Cost-Effective Quality Control: Managing the Quality and Productivity of Analytical Processes

Related books on this topic from AACC Press

Quality Assurance in Health Care: A Critical Appraisal of Clinical Chemistry
Royden N. Rand, Russell J. Eilers, Noel S. Lawton, and Alan Broughton, editors

The Clinical Laboratory in the New Era: Quality, Cost, and Diagnostic Demands
Edward W. Bermes, Jr., editor

Cost-Effective Quality Control: Managing the Quality and Productivity of Analytical Processes

James O. Westgard and Patricia L. Barry

With a Foreword by Royden N. Rand

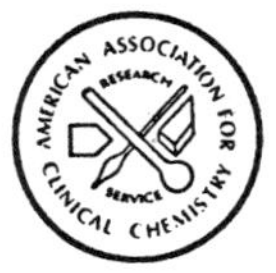

AACC Press
American Association for Clinical Chemistry
2029 K Street, NW
Washington, DC 20006

James O. Westgard, Ph.D., is Professor, Department of Pathology and Laboratory Medicine, Department of Medicine, University of Wisconsin Medical School; Affiliate Faculty, Medical Technology Program, School of Allied Health Professions; Associate Director of Clinical Laboratories–Quality Assurance, University of Wisconsin Hospital and Clinics, Madison, WI.

Patricia L. Barry, B.S., MT (ASCP), is Quality Assurance Supervisor, Clinical Laboratories, University of Wisconsin Hospital and Clinics, Madison, WI.

Dedicated to Russell J. Eilers, M.D., 1925–1985, who recognized the potential applications of industrial quality management in clinical laboratories and health-care organizations.

Library of Congress Cataloging in Publication Data

Westgard, James O., 1941–
Cost-effective quality control.

Includes bibliographies and index.
1. Pathological laboratories—Quality control—Cost effectiveness. 2. Diagnosis, Laboratory—Quality control—Cost effectiveness. I. Barry, Patricia L., 1948– . II. Title. [DNLM: 1. Cost Benefit Analysis —methods. 2. Laboratories—organization & administration. 3. Quality Control. QY 23 W528c]
RB36.3.Q34W47 1986 362.1'77'068 86–7933

ISBN 0–915274–35–3

Printed in the United States of America

Third Printing 1992

CONTENTS

FOREWORD

The advent of DRGs (Diagnosis Related Groups) has caused the clinical laboratory to become a cost center. Although the key role of laboratory data in the diagnosis and care of patients is not challenged, significant efforts to control laboratory costs and to increase revenue are underway.

In recent years, the concepts involved in quality management or total quality control have been advanced for developing cost-effective operations in American industry. Underlying the work of Juran, Deming, Feigenbaum, and others is the postulate that comprehensive attention to quality by management leads to improved productivity by eliminating rework and improving customer satisfaction. Even though money and effort must be invested to control quality, successful implementation of total quality control will, as has been demonstrated by these and other authors, produce a decrease of total costs. The fundamental ideas involved in quality management are well reviewed in Chapter 1.

Eilers, in 1975,[1] was the first to urge the application of quality management principles to the clinical laboratory, in an attempt to apply the principles developed by Feigenbaum. In 1976, the Liaison Committee of the American Association for Clinical Chemistry and the College of American Pathologists recommended that the two organizations sponsor a national conference to promote the concepts and principles of "total quality control," as outlined in Feigenbaum's textbook.[2] In 1979, Feigenbaum delivered the keynote address for the conference.

Since publication of the proceedings from the conference,[3] there has been little, if any, further development of the quality-management principles in clinical laboratories. Thus, the appearance of this book from Dr. Westgard and Ms. Barry is a welcome renewal of the principles and their application in clinical laboratories, as foreseen by Dr. Eilers and the AACC–CAP Liaison Committee.

The underlying assumptions of the book are:

1. Regardless of resource limitations, the quality of clinical laboratory measurements must be sustained or improved.
2. The principles of quality management can be applied in the laboratory to achieve "cost-effective quality control."

Many of us were brought up to think of quality control as comprising

---

[1] Eilers RJ. Quality assurance in health care: missions, goals, activities. Clin Chem 1975; 21:1357–67.

[2] Feigenbaum AV. Total quality control, 3rd ed. New York: McGraw-Hill, 1983.

[3] Rand RN, Eilers RJ, Lawson NS, Broughton A, Eds. Quality assurance in health care: a critical appraisal of clinical chemistry. Washington, DC: American Association for Clinical Chemistry, 1980.

assays of one or more controls and drawing Shewhart and Levey–Jennings charts. Often the data were reviewed only monthly; in fact, nothing was really controlled. Westgard and Barry make clear that one must start with quality goals and then develop a strategy for control, based on the principles elaborated in this book.

There should be no mistake about the real nature of quality control; it demands thorough understanding of the underlying mathematics. I suggest that readers start by examining Chapter 1 (Managing quality and productivity), Chapter 2 (Analytical processes—the production processes in clinical laboratories), and Chapter 7 (Selecting and designing cost-effective quality-control procedures). These three chapters give an excellent overview of the subject matter and will prepare you for the more technical material presented in the other chapters. However, all of the chapters can be understood by anyone in this field after appropriate study.

Westgard and Barry succeed admirably in meeting their objectives, for which I congratulate them. There can be no subject more important these days than maintaining quality services while facing severe cost pressures.

Royden N. Rand, Ph.D.
Past-President, AACC

PREFACE

This book, *Cost-Effective Quality Control,* is about managing the quality and productivity of analytical processes in clinical laboratories. It focuses on the selection and design of statistical control procedures, but it is not a traditional text about statistical quality control. There is no attempt to provide comprehensive coverage of the many statistical control procedures that could be applied, though some selected examples are presented of control procedures that are practical in clinical laboratories. The book is intended for practitioners of quality control—clinical chemists, clinical pathologists, and medical technologists—the analysts and managers in clinical laboratories.

Chapter 1 (Managing quality and productivity) is an introduction to industrial quality management and provides the basis for defining cost-effective quality control as the "use of a control procedure that maximizes both the quality and productivity of an analytical process." This definition is central to the approach in the rest of the book.

Chapter 2 (Analytical processes—the production processes in clinical laboratories) is background material for understanding how an analytical process is established, how quality specifications guide the evaluation of a measurement procedure and the selection and design of a control procedure, and how statistical quality control is practiced in clinical laboratories.

Chapter 3 (Characterizing the quality of statistical control procedures) describes how a control procedure can be evaluated and compared with other control procedures. Chapter 4 (Improving quality control by the use of multi-rule control procedures) applies the concepts in a detailed example of a multi-rule control procedure, evaluating the performance of this control procedure and comparing it with the performance of other control procedures that are commonly used in clinical laboratories.

Chapters 5 and 6 (Predicting the quality and productivity of an analytical process) illustrate how quality and productivity are affected by different quality-control procedures. With the aid of quality–productivity planning models, a manager or analyst can select and design control procedures on the basis of their cost-effectiveness.

Chapter 7 (Selecting and designing cost-effective quality-control procedures) provides a summary of the principles for cost-effective quality control, some guidelines for developing control procedures, and some strategies for implementation. A glossary of terms is found at the end of the book, including a glossary of control rules. Appendices provide information on the performance of many commonly used control procedures and descriptions of spreadsheet programs for performing some of the calculations described in Chapters 3 through 6.

Some readers may find it useful to start with Chapter 7 to gain an overview of the material and approach, then read the background material in Chapters 1 and 2 before studying the more quantitative presentations in Chapters 3 through 6.

Cost-Effective Quality Control has evolved from quality-control workshops presented at scientific meetings. The book became a project in the Educational Resources Subcommittee of the American Association for Clinical Chemistry, where it was actively supported and promoted by Edward W. Bermes, Jr., chairman of the Education Committee.

The book draws much from past work with Carl-Henric de Verdier, Torgny Groth, and Torsten Aronsson, collaborators from Uppsala University in Sweden, who have been involved in many of the technical papers that are cited. Torgny has been a full partner in the development of the concepts and ideas presented here, and developed the computer simulation program that has allowed us to study the performance of control procedures. More recently, Per Hyltoft Petersen, a collaborator from Odense University in Denmark, has contributed to these ideas, particularly the development of the models for predicting the performance of analytical processes. These associations have been rich and rewarding, personally and professionally.

We have also been fortunate to have associates at the University of Wisconsin who understood our interests in quality control. Frank Larson has made it possible for us to dedicate our efforts to quality-assurance activities. Arthur Eggert has provided computer support for design tools and application programs, and has also critiqued the manuscript for the book. Tim Kramer and Tom Blankenheim have supported the simulation program; Elliot Chandler and Ken Emmerich have provided the plotting programs for preparing the power-function graphs. Neill Carey, Carl Garber, George Cembrowski, Ronald Laessig, Anne Sullivan, and Marian Hunt have all contributed to the ideas presented here.

We thank David Plaut and Roy Rand for their review of the manuscript and their many helpful comments. The readability of the book has been greatly improved by Virginia Marcum, who has edited the text and clarified our thoughts.

The people who have helped the most, though, are Joan, Kristin, and Sten, and Rick and Erica, who have tolerated our obsession with this project and given up many hours of family time as we struggled to complete the writing. Without them, none of this would have been possible or worthwhile.

James O. Westgard
Patricia L. Barry

CHAPTER 1

Managing Quality and Productivity

The future success of health-care organizations—even their survival—may well depend on their ability to improve quality and productivity. Higher-quality services will be necessary to satisfy patients and maintain a share of the market; higher productivity will be necessary for financial success. Organizations having problems with quality and productivity simply will not stay in business.

Who is responsible for an organization's problems with quality and productivity? According to experts on industrial quality, management is. "[The] cause of quality-control problems might be managers—not workers" (*1*). Because improving quality requires reshaping attitudes throughout the organization, management has to take the initiative. New approaches for managing quality have to be implemented.

In this introduction to "quality management," the discussion of quality and productivity and their relationship to cost is drawn from quality-management approaches developed for managing quality in industry. The approaches recommended by four industrial experts—W. Edwards Deming, J. M. Juran, Armand V. Feigenbaum, and Philip B. Crosby—are presented and a list of educational materials for further pursuit of this subject is included at the end of the chapter.

"Quality management" has broad implications for the management and quality-assurance programs of hospitals and clinical laboratories, as will be evident in this introduction. However, it is our purpose in the rest of this book to apply the concepts to the use of quality control in clinical laboratories. Quality control is a tool for the technical management of analytical processes, i.e., a tool for managing the quality and productivity of analytical processes.

Introduction to Quality Management

Given that whole books have been written on the subject of quality management (see list at end of chapter), we have used a question-and-answer format to focus on important issues for understanding how the cost-effectiveness of quality-control procedures relates to the quality and productivity of analytical processes.

What is "quality management"?

"Quality management" refers to a management approach in which quality is first in importance in management activities and decision making. The best-known advocate of this approach is W. Edwards Deming, an American statistician credited with helping Japanese industry rebuild and excel in the competitive international market. Deming (*2*) stresses that improved quality leads to improved productivity by eliminating "rework"—that is, the need to do things over because they were done wrong the first time and the quality was not satisfactory. Improved productivity leads to lower costs because time and materials are saved by the elimination of rework. Lower costs, in turn, provide a price advantage and a competitive position, thus permitting an organization to stay in business and provide jobs. According to Deming, quality means jobs in today's competitive environment, and the unemployment in some American industries is an indictment of past management practices (*3*).

Figure 1-1 illustrates this concept of quality management. Quality is the most important factor for the economic well-being of a company; it is more important for the company to achieve quality than to achieve

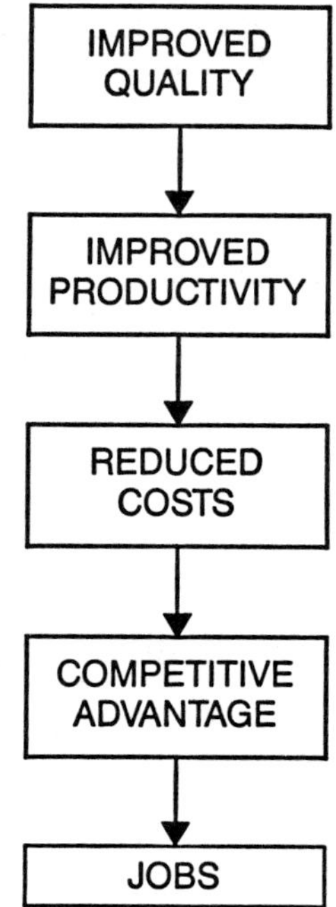

Fig. 1-1. Strategy for quality management

numbers (volume of production). Past management approaches, aimed at increasing production to reduce per-unit cost through increased volume, have given secondary consideration to the quality of the product.

Several different names have been applied to this management approach. Of the four leading industrial experts on quality, Deming and Juran seem to prefer "quality improvement." Feigenbaum, as well as Japanese industry, uses the term "total quality control." Crosby uses "quality management." All these names are understood in industry to refer to this approach, but to managers and analysts in clinical laboratories, the term "quality management" probably most clearly indicates the principle of "quality first in management" and differentiates this approach from the current practices in "quality assurance" and "quality control."

Why is the management of quality important?

Health-care providers in the United States have entered a new competitive era. Changes in government reimbursement policies have limited the amount of money that is paid for medical care. Payment of flat fees, based on Diagnostic Related Groups (DRGs), has effectively limited hospital and laboratory charges (*4*). Support of Health Maintenance Organizations and similar prepaid medical plans has created new health-care organizations to compete with traditional providers. The new "competitive marketplace" puts pressure on a provider not only to reduce the costs of products and services but also, and at the same time, to improve their quality, to maintain or increase the share of the market. The effect on clinical laboratories is that performing more tests no longer guarantees more revenue or increased resources to support new tests and services. In addition, the quality of the laboratory's testing services and their usefulness to the physician and patient must be at least maintained and, in many cases, improved.

"Cost-effectiveness" has become a major concern of managers. When this idea is translated into practice, the emphasis is more often on reducing costs than increasing effectiveness. "Cost" seems to be more easily understood and more directly measured and controlled. "Effectiveness" is both difficult to understand and measure. Effectiveness relates to quality, and managers generally seem to believe that it is difficult, if not impossible, to measure quality. It is important for managers to learn that, to the contrary, quality can be measured.

In controlling costs, most managers recognize that increased productivity will be a key to the future financial success and survival of health-care organizations (*5*). The impact of improved productivity on cost is easy to understand. Costs will be reduced when fewer resources are required to provide a product or service. But what will be the impact on quality? The general attitude seems to be that "ultimate" quality can not be achieved, given the need to control costs; standards for quality must, however, be kept as high as possible, so that, with luck, quality will not suffer too much under cost control.

Efforts to reduce costs could compromise quality; for example, a decrease in laboratory staffing could mean longer turnaround times for reporting test results, causing delays in treatment and affecting a patient's outcome. The turnaround time for laboratory tests is an issue of quality, but it may not be given fair consideration with the issue of cost because it is not as well understood. Little is taught in business and management about quality and how to improve it, in contrast to what is taught about costs and how to control them.

Managers of health-care organizations must start to understand the relationships between quality, productivity, and cost, and must learn how to manage quality. American industry has learned some hard lessons in this regard, and health-care providers should profit from those experiences. Faced with international competition, American industries are beginning to develop new management approaches to provide better quality at lower cost. "Quality First" has become the motto: quality is the primary issue; productivity and cost are secondary. However, proper management of quality can provide gains in productivity and reductions in cost.

Industrial experiences have demonstrated that quality and cost do not have to be trade-offs. According to Philip B. Crosby, another industrial expert in quality management, quality is free: it is the *lack* of quality that costs (*6*). Both high quality and low cost can be achieved if management understands its responsibility for quality improvement and implements a quality-management program.

What does "quality" really mean?

The word "quality" is so widely used and apparently so well understood that it is seldom defined, even in hospital accreditation documents that outline requirements for quality assurance (*7*). Crosby (*8*) perhaps best explains the difficulty in understanding quality. "Quality," he says, "has much in common with sex. Everyone is for it. (Under certain conditions, of course.) Everyone feels they understand it. (Even though they wouldn't want to explain it.) Everyone thinks execution is only a matter of following natural inclination. (After all, we do get along somehow.) And, of course, most people feel that all problems in these areas are caused by other people. (If only they would take time to do things right.)"

The problem is that people don't understand quality in a quantitative way. Quality is generally thought to mean excellence or goodness. But excellence and goodness are not measurable. The lack of a widely accepted operational definition of quality is the major reason why people find quality difficult to measure.

Industry has learned that quality means "conformance to the requirements of users or customers." This operational definition draws from Crosby's definition of quality as "conformance to requirements" (*9*), Juran's emphasis on "fitness for use" (*10*), and the American Society for Quality Control's definition of quality as "the totality of features and characteristics of a product or service that bear on its ability to satisfy given needs" (*11*). The quality of laboratory tests and services is related to the needs of its users or customers, who are patients, or physicians or nurses acting on the behalf of patients.

We use the term "quality requirements" to describe the many features and characteristics of a laboratory testing service that would bear on its ability to satisfy its users. Table 1-1 lists quality requirements for laboratory tests and services.

When quality is defined in terms of requirements, the quality of analytical testing services can be measured because conformance to the requirements can be determined. For example, if a quality requirement is a turnaround time of 60 min or less for a test result (requirement L in Table 1-1), then the turnaround time can be measured and a determination made as to whether the requirement is satisfied. For each of the quality requirements outlined in Table 1-1, measurements can be identified to determine whether the requirements are satisfied. Thus, the quality of analytical testing services can be monitored and evaluated.

For further detailed discussion of quality, including definitions of related terms such as "imperfection," "nonconformance," and "defect," see the article by Freund (*12*). He concludes that "quality is a composite concept. The relative importance of characteristics and features varies over time as well as among users. Needs, or perceptions of needs, change. Thus the quality of a product or service cannot be taken for granted. It is a dynamic force."

Why does quality take priority over productivity?

Productivity is more readily measured than quality because more work has been done on productivity measurements. Productivity is determined by measuring the amount of product produced and the amount of resources consumed; a ratio of "output" to "input," its units depend on the measurements chosen.

Deming cautions against putting too much emphasis on the measurement of productivity. He acknowledges the usefulness of such measurements for comparing productivity, past and present, that of your organization and others, etc., but he also points out that the efforts to measure productivity do not themselves lead to any improvements in productiv-

Table 1-1. Quality Requirements for a Laboratory Testing Service

A. Qualified staff, with appropriate education, experience, and in-service training, adequate in number to meet the service demands and supported with the resources necessary to deliver the requested tests and services.

B. Adequate facilities, including instruments and equipment, dependable sources of supply for reagents and materials, adequate stocks with proper storage to maintain continuity, to deliver the requested tests and services.

C. Availability of appropriate tests, selected for their diagnostic sensitivity and specificity to provide medically useful information.

D. Availability of diverse tests and testing protocols, to provide the scope, variety, and cost-effectiveness required for the patient population to be treated.

E. Availability of appropriate services based on the needs to acquire specimens, perform testing, and report results.

F. Adequate and reliable specimens, correctly requested and scheduled, of proper material and sample size, obtained at approprate times for both the convenience of the patient and the validity of the tests, collected in proper specimen containers, with correct patient identification and proper labeling, from patients properly prepared and correctly identified.

G. Prompt delivery of specimens, stored properly during transport.

H. Proper specimen processing, including evaluation of specimen integrity and suitability for the requested tests, with samples stored properly after processing, to assure the stability of the analyte to be measured.

I. Proper identification, aliquoting, and distribution of samples, including those sent to outside laboratories.

J. Analytical testing available to fit the demands of use, whether routine service daily, priority service with specified time needs, or 24-h emergency service.

K. Appropriate analytical quality, including analytical sensitivity (detection limit, absence of false negatives), specificity (freedom from interfering materials, absence of false positives), precision, and accuracy, as verified initially by method-evaluation studies and routinely by statistical quality-control procedures.

L. Turnaround times to meet the needs for the specific tests requested, order status of the test request, and clinical service making the request.

M. Reporting formats, appropriate for both laboratory and hospital computer reports, meeting the needs for emergency testing, for test results exceeding "alert values," and for routine testing, with timely daily and cumulative reports identifying abnormal results, interfering substances, and, when appropriate, analytical conditions.

N. Reference ranges, verified for appropriate populations, including subpopulations selected by sex and age.

O. Proper interpretation of test results for appropriate patient care.

P. Reasonable costs for the testing services provided.

Q. Communication mechanisms for providing the information necessary to utilize laboratory services effectively, to provide feedback from users or customers when quality is not satisfactory, and to notify users or customers when problems occur.

Source: Clinical Laboratories Quality Assurance Plan, University of Wisconsin Hospital, Madison, WI.

ity. "Measures of productivity are like statistics on accidents: they tell you all about the number of accidents in the home, on the road, and at the work place, but they do not tell you how to reduce the frequency of accidents" (*13*).

Productivity can be improved by increasing the output (the numerator) or decreasing the input (the denominator). However, one problem with emphasizing productivity over quality is that productivity can be increased by producing a product having unsatisfactory quality. [There usually is no distinction made between the production of "good" and "bad" product.] Another problem is that attempts to improve productivity may focus on curtailing resources without improving the production process, therefore precipitating the production of more "bad" product.

By emphasizing quality over productivity, efforts are first directed at maximizing "good" output, which increases the numerator. These efforts will also reduce waste of resources, which decreases the denominator. Improved quality provides real gains in production (output), and at the same time provides savings in resources (input).

There is an established system for measuring productivity in clinical laboratories—the College of American Pathologists (CAP) Laboratory Workload Recording Method (*14*). "Output" for an analytical procedure is measured in workload units (minutes) and is calculated by counting the number of tests or items (standards, controls, repeats, etc.) performed per procedure, then multiplying by a workload factor or "unit value" (average number of minutes of staff time required to perform all steps necessary to complete the procedure once). CAP provides a detailed manual, listing hundreds of analytical methods and the unit values assigned based on time-and-motion studies. The work units for all tests performed in the laboratory are determined and then summed to provide the total "output" for the laboratory, expressed as total work units (minutes).

"Input" is measured by the number of hours of staffing required to produce that output. Productivity is calculated by dividing the total work units (minutes) by the hours of staffing, and is expressed in units of minutes per hour. Staffing hours can be calculated in terms of the total hours paid, hours worked (paid hours minus vacation, sick leave, etc.), or hours with other specified deductions (hours for teaching, in-service training, etc.); therefore, productivity can actually have several different meanings and may be expressed in numerically different values for identical tasks.

The CAP measure of productivity does not distinguish between production of good or bad test results (product). "Rework," repeat analyses, is credited as additional work. In industry, that part of the production facilities devoted to rework is called the "hidden plant"—a plant existing within a plant to correct the errors and mistakes made in the course of production. Similarly, there is a "hidden laboratory" within every clinical laboratory. The repeat work is credited as productive work, although the analytical capacity of the laboratory is actually being reduced. Feigenbaum estimates that, in industry, productivity can be improved by 20% to 30% by eliminating the hidden plant (*15*).

A different measure of productivity that can be calculated from the CAP workload data is the "test yield" of each analytical process (*16*). The number of patients' samples submitted for analysis is divided by the total number of tests required to produce results for those patients (patients' samples, standards, controls, repeats). For example, if obtaining results of a single test for 140 patients' samples requires performing a total of 200 analytical tests, the analytical process has a 70% test yield. That means 30% of the tests performed by this analytical process do not directly provide patients' results. Some of these tests are performed for calibration and control, which are important functions for preventing errors and detecting them when they occur. Others are repeats due to problems with the analytical method, e.g., samples in analytical runs that are "out of control" and must be reanalyzed. Such repeats represent waste; if their number could be decreased, the productivity or test yield of the analytical process would be improved. "Test yield" is a useful measure of the productivity of an analytical process because it does not credit "bad" product or repeat analyses as productive work. Furthermore, it may provide a more realistic estimate of costs, because data on the actual cost per test should consider the amount of process output that is wasted. In later chapters, the concept of test yield is used to evaluate the effect of different designs of quality control on the resulting quality and productivity of an analytical process.

What "cost" is really important?

Cost must be considered in broad terms. Feigenbaum (*17*) introduced the concept of "quality-costs" in the manufacturing industries in the 1950s in an effort to get management to understand the costs of quality for the organization as a whole. Quality-costs include the costs associated with achieving satisfactory quality, as well as the costs associated with producing products and services of unsatisfactory quality.

As shown in Figure 1-2, the costs for satisfactory quality can be described as the "costs of conformance" and include "prevention costs" incurred to prevent defects and nonconformities, and "appraisal costs" incurred to measure and control quality via inspection, audit, and statistical quality control. The costs for unsatisfactory quality are "costs of nonconformance," which include "internal failure costs" incurred due to scrap and rework and "external failure costs" incurred due to cus-

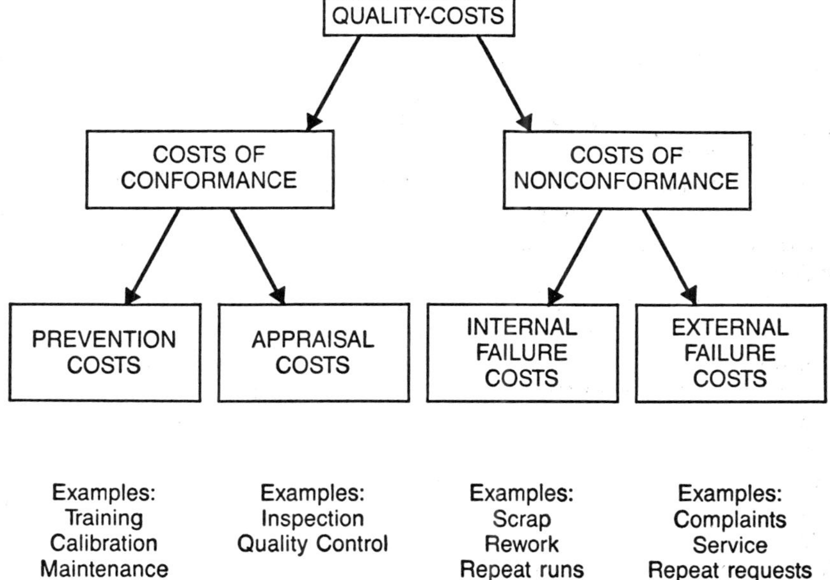

Fig. 1-2. The costs of quality (conformance) and the costs of lack of quality (nonconformance)

tomer complaints and customer service. The terms scrap, rework, customer complaints, and customer service are easily understood with regard to manufacturing industries, but they also apply to the discarded results, repeated analyses, repeated requests, and additional requests for testing in a clinical laboratory.

In assessing costs for quality, it is easy to consider only the prevention or appraisal costs because those costs show up directly in departmental budgets. In clinical laboratories, for example, one can easily assess the costs for statistical quality control without any thought to the costs incurred if such control were inadequate. Laboratory records show the costs for purchases of control materials and the time and expense of analyzing those materials. Costs for inadequate control, however, aren't found in the records of the laboratory because they are incurred by other departments when patients are treated on the basis on unreliable test results or inadequate service.

Therefore, a broad view of costs is necessary to consider the costs to an organization as a whole, rather than just the costs in individual departments. Cost reductions in one department may cause increases in another department, and even lead to an overall loss for the organization as a whole. Unfortunately, failure costs generally go unrecognized because they do not show up as line items on any departmental budget;

the additional time, effort, and materials involved are added to other line items.

Golden (*18*) argues for this broader view of costs when discussing the need for cost cutters to adopt a more "holistic" approach. He states that "the primary purpose of laboratories is to provide physicians with information for making diagnoses and monitoring therapy. Under DRGs, minimizing average length of stay per patient is highly desirable." Health-care providers analyzing costs must consider the importance of laboratory service in contributing to the earlier discharge of patients.

The potential cost savings from prompt laboratory service can be illustrated by considering the failure costs associated with the turnaround time of a test. For example, a slow response to a request for determination of creatine kinase isoenzymes could cause a patient to remain an extra day in an intensive-care unit. The additional expense to the hospital may be $1000 more than if the patient were in a non-intensive-care unit. Or, a slow response in determining bacterial sensitivities could cause an extra day of hospitalization before treatment with the proper antibiotic, adding $600 to the costs for treatment of that patient. If slow responses of the laboratory were to cause only one additional patient day for every day of operation in a year, the failure costs would be nearly a quarter of a million dollars (365 times $600 equals $219 000).

In an effort to get employees to understand the consequences of inadequate or unsatisfactory services, some hospitals have gone so far as to offer patients a rebate of $10 for each meal that was not satisfactory and $20 for each act of discourtesy on the part of a staff member (*19*). Failure-costs, then, are understandable as real costs, in monetary units. The rebate policy makes good sense if one considers the potential losses from a patient who won't return because of poor service, and from other patients who choose other hospitals because of word-of-mouth complaints by a dissatisfied patient. From industrial studies on customer satisfaction, Feigenbaum determined that a satisfied customer tells eight others, whereas a dissatisfied customer tells 22 others (*15*). The bad advertising from a dissatisfied customer far outweighs the benefits of good advertising by a satisfied customer.

The concept of quality-costs is not without precedent in health-care organizations; in fact, quality-costs are analogous to similar costs in "risk management." Health-care providers in the United States, aware of the potentially large costs resulting from medical malpractice suits, generally have developed specific risk-management programs to prevent the occurrence of such suits and thereby limit the costs to the organization. They must learn to apply the same ideas in a widespread quality-management program.

Can improved quality really reduce costs?

The magnitude of the savings from quality improvements could be tremendous. In manufacturing industries, Feigenbaum has documented quality-costs as 10% to 30% of gross sales (*15*). Two-thirds of these costs are failure costs; if quality were properly managed, 5% to 20% of gross receipts could be saved. In other words, as much as 20% of present gross sales could become profit, without any increase in sales or market share. In service industries, quality-costs may be as high as 35% of operating costs (*20*).

Crosby's conclusion that "quality is free" is based on his knowledge of the magnitude of quality-costs and the large portion that is failure costs. Improved quality can lead to reduced costs because of the amount of money that is already being wasted by producing goods and services of unsatisfactory quality. It takes an investment in quality improvement to secure the savings, but the return on investment may be higher than any other money-making opportunity available to the organization.

How is quality achieved?

The system for achieving quality is prevention. That means careful planning to avoid problems, rather than responding to problems and correcting them after they occur. Problems must be solved permanently, not just temporarily for today's production run. When problems are prevented, quality improves, productivity increases, costs are reduced, and the company's competitive position improves.

Crosby's definition of quality management clearly focuses on prevention (*21*). "Quality management is a systematic way of guaranteeing that organized activities happen the way they are planned. It is a management discipline concerned with preventing problems from occurring by creating the attitudes and controls that make prevention possible."

He uses analogies to ballet and hockey to contrast quality management with the style of management practiced in many organizations (*22*). In ballet, there is a carefully rehearsed plan and each performance happens the same way every time. All of the performers know their jobs and do them in a carefully coordinated manner to achieve quality. In hockey, all of the players know their positions, but once the puck is dropped, every performance is a new and unique experience. All work hard and to the best of their abilities—which sometimes is enough to achieve the desired quality, but not always.

What is the goal for quality?

Deming talks about constancy of purpose being necessary for continual quality improvement. Juran describes the need for an annual ongoing quality-improvement program, not just a one-time program. Crosby describes the goal as being "zero defects," meaning that no mistakes or errors should be tolerated. The point is that quality is a way of life. The efforts never stop, though they may start over again and again. Organizations must strive continually to improve the quality of their products and services if they expect to remain competitive.

In presenting the concept of zero defects, Crosby acknowledges that most people react negatively to the idea because they think zero defects is impossible (*23*). Indeed, people are conditioned to believe that some mistakes or errors are inevitable. To counter that belief, he cites an example of an almost universal expectation of zero defects: Will you accept an error in your paycheck 5% percent of the time? Not likely!

In presenting the concept of zero defects to medical personnel, Gambino (*24*) poses a similar example. How many dropped babies are acceptable in the nursery? Obviously the answer is zero; such mistakes cannot be tolerated. Even though there may have been some incidents from which one could establish an average or norm, performing up to the norm is not an acceptable goal; the only acceptable goal is zero defects.

Zero defects is a goal that can be used in a simple way. For example, in a report of the number of incidents in which test results do not meet the requirements for turnaround time—say, 10 incidents out of 10 000—the numbers can be presented as 10 incidents, instead of 0.10%. Presenting the results in absolute numbers, rather than as a percentage, puts emphasis on the number of times the problems occur and makes it more difficult to disregard the problems just because they are a small percentage.

Who is responsible for quality?

Experience in industry has led to what is known as the 85/15 rule (quoted by Juran, Deming, and others): 85% of the problems are system or process problems that can be solved only by management; only the remaining 15% of the problems can be solved by workers. Quality is therefore a management problem. Most improvements require changing the system or process, which means changing the way things are done. Only management has the power to make these changes; therefore, quality improvement can occur only if there is commitment by management.

Management must provide the leadership if quality improvement is to become the guiding strategy for an organization. Top management must take the time to understand quality, to learn how to manage quality, and to be involved personally. If management does not take this active role, then most problems (85%) will not be solved. Workers' efforts through "quality circles" and similar peer-group teams can solve only about 15% of the problems, which explains the limited success of quality-circle programs when management does not understand its responsibility. An important difference in Japan's success with quality circles has been that management commitment and participation came first (with Deming's and Juran's insistence), before the development of worker-participative approaches such as quality circles.

Case studies illustrate the importance of management leadership. For example, two years after starting a quality-improvement program in a medical manufacturing company, Mead (*25*) described his experience as follows:

> I have seen . . . that if I change directions, the people around me also change. If I push for quality, they respond with quality. If I push for numbers [production], they respond with numbers. I have had to come to grips with this fact: I am the leader, and my employees follow the direction I set. American workers want to do a good job but management often refuses to give them the tools and support to do it. Very few problems at our company in the last 20 months—rejects, complaints, late deliveries, or other related problems—can't be traced back to a system problem. As Deming says, '85% of the problems within a company are system problems and only top management has the power to change the system.' The responsibility for the slipping U.S. position in the world's industrial marketplace falls squarely on the shoulders of management. If management got us here, only management can take us back.

What exactly is management commitment to quality?

The best explanation may be that offered by Lammi (*26*):

> Quality commitment is not just a speech that declares one to be for good quality. Everyone is for good quality. It is not the showing of videotapes that show what can happen if we don't have good quality. It is not a pep talk that urges employees to pay attention to good quality.
>
> Quality commitment is not increasing inspection to sort out bad production. It is not making rework a permanent part of the process. It does not mean trouble-shooting problems after they occur. It does not mean finding the cause of every defect and assigning the fault to the workforce.
>
> Quality commitment is not a public relations program with empty action items. It is not a low priority item to be addressed whenever all other work is done. It is not a program for filling in time by having quality meetings with the workforce. It is not verbal support for improving quality without any personal effort.
>
> What quality commitment is, is the planning and implementation of a program of action for continuous improvement of quality. It is the education and training of people to do their jobs better.
>
> It is the forming of problem-solving teams made up of cross sections of various disciplines to tackle chronic problems.
>
> Quality commitment is the use of statistics to control processes and to indicate problem areas.

It is the breaking down of barriers between departments in order to work together for a common solution.

Quality commitment is listening to suggestions for improvement made by people doing their jobs and the prompt implementation of those improvements accepted by management.

Quality commitment is the provision of tools to workers to do their best work, the allowance of time to do the job right, and the recognition of good work.

Quality commitment is the commitment of all resources to improve the processes.

How is quality management implemented?

Once management understands quality and is committed to quality improvement, there needs to be widespread education and training, first for top and middle managers, then for supervisors, and finally for workers. The educational efforts are ongoing to keep pace with changing needs. Several different training programs may be used, as outlined by MacKinnon (*27*). Top management could start with a program by Crosby to understand quality, establish a quality policy, and organize the quality-improvement effort. Another program on project management and problem solving could use Juran's training materials. Additional programs on statistical quality control and industrial engineering techniques may be necessary later on.

Because quality improvement occurs on a project-by-project basis by identifying and solving problems, the education and training must set the stage for developing group problem-solving approaches. The objective is to have all employees in the organization participate, to take advantage of their knowledge of the processes, their insights into the problems, and their solutions.

Problem-solving teams are formed to formally encourage cooperation and teamwork. A *project team* is a small group of people who are appointed by management to solve a specific quality problem. Also called "quality teams," "quality-improvement teams," or "corrective action teams," the development of teams and teamwork takes time and effort. John A. Young, the president of Hewlett-Packard and the chairman of the President's Commission on Industrial Competitiveness, has outlined the following characteristics of successful quality teams (*28*) [bracketed material added for emphasis]:

> First, quality teams need to be closely integrated into strategic business goals. [Teams aren't viewed as ancillary, but as vehicles for pursuing major strategic objectives.]
>
> Second, managers must "own" the teams as a vehicle to achieve those goals. [Ownership here means personal involvement, not just support.]
>
> Third, the teams must be thoroughly equipped with the skills and tools

needed to get the job done. [This includes training in problem solving, statistics, teambuilding, and process analysis.]

The final requirement for successful teamwork has to be an organization's management style. Do managers view their employees as their customers? Are they good listeners? Do they encourage honest feedback? Are they willing to compromise? Do they value consensus? Are they willing to invest the time it takes to create it? These and scores of other questions reflect the vast gulf between management theory and practice. They also reflect how essential it is that managers model the very behavior they want to encourage. . . . Teamwork is more easily praised than practiced.

For more widespread involvement and participation of workers, quality circles provide another kind of a team. A *quality circle* "is a group of people who voluntarily meet together on a regular basis to identify, analyze, and solve quality and other problems in their area" (*29*). Circles differ from project teams in several ways: their primary purpose is human relations, with quality improvement being secondary—nonetheless, they are essential for solving the 15% of problems that management cannot eliminate (remember the 85/15 rule); the members volunteer, instead of being appointed by management; the members tend to be peers and workers, rather than managers and supervisors; circles generally operate within a department, not across departments, and therefore focus on intradepartmental rather than interdepartmental problems; and they are standing or continuous teams that meet regularly, rather than ad hoc teams (*30*). Circles provide workers with an opportunity to participate in the decision-making process and provide an effective mechanism for dealing with issues regarding the quality of work life. Because satisfied workers will more readily produce products and services that result in satisfied customers, quality circles can be an important addition to project teams for implementing a quality-management program.

With teamwork and employee participation in identification and resolution of problems, quality becomes everyone's job. Everyone is responsible for improving the process to achieve quality. Because this usually requires major changes in management style and organizational culture, the implementation of quality management takes a long time, typically three to five years.

Is quality management applicable to "service" industries?

Whatever their mission, companies are organizations of people. Quality management is concerned with planning the activities of those people to achieve the mission of the company, whether it is a car assembly plant, a bank, an insurance company, a government department, a hospital, or a clinical laboratory. There are many examples of applications of quality management to service industries (*31*). With the transition of American industry from manufacturing to service, quality management will be extensively applied to service organizations.

Aren't health-care organizations different?

In providing health care, the quality of services is more critically dependent on the performance of every individual in the organization. The expectations and requirements of the customer are higher than for most other businesses. The need for quality management is even greater.

The closest analogy to the workings of a health-care organization is "just-in-time" (JIT) industrial production (*32*). "Just-in-time" means that a component is produced or delivered just in time for assembly. There is no inventory of materials, because inventory itself represents waste in materials, space, time, etc. JIT forces the highest level of quality because there is no room for mistakes or errors. If an item or service is not satisfactory, the whole process comes to a stop. JIT demands quality.

In health-care organizations, every patient is an individual with special problems that must be sorted out (diagnosed). The process requires highly individualized treatment. On the basis of one finding, another procedure is required—now, immediately, just-in-time for diagnosis and treatment. The delivery of health care demands quality.

How do practices of quality management compare with practices of quality control?

Organizations faced with the demands of JIT recognize that the old methods for managing quality via quality control must be replaced with a quality-management approach. Sepehri (*33*) contrasts the new and old styles (images) for managing quality in Table 1-2 and reviews and summarizes the differences between quality control ("old image") and quality management ("new image").

Is "quality management" practiced in hospitals and clinical laboratories?

The management of quality in hospitals and clinical laboratories is carried out under the name of "quality assurance." The American Society for Quality Control (ASQC) defines quality assurance as "all those planned or systematic actions necessary to provide adequate confidence that a product or service will satisfy given needs" (*11*). The definition specifies products and services, and clinical laboratories provide both: a product in the form of a test result, and services in obtaining specimens and reporting results appropriately.

Quality assurance, as used by the Joint Commission on Accreditation for Hospitals (*7*), refers to "an ongoing program designed to objec-

Table 1-2. Managing Quality by Control ("Old Image") vs Approach of Quality Management ("New Image")

Old image	New image
Low quality is caused by low performance of people. Automation is the key to higher quality.	Low quality is caused by poor management of people. Respect for people is the key to higher quality.
Loss of work ethic causes poor quality in the U.S. The Japanese maintain a quality edge due to their ethical and cultural values.	American workers, when properly managed, are as good as or better than any others, particularly in their commitment to jobs.
Some defects are acceptable. [Products] are accepted if they meet minimum average quality standards.	Zero defects is the goal. There is not a minimum average acceptable quality. All units should be free of defects.
Inspect for product problems regularly, then rework. Rework is done at a later and separate stage.	Inspect for process problems, and fix problems so that they do not recur. Any repair work is done on the line with no delay.
Higher quality means higher costs and therefore lower profits. Quality is expensive and a burden to manufacturing.	Higher quality is a means to higher profits. Quality is the goal; it is not a burden to manufacturing.
Quality is inspected into the product. Nonconforming units are continuously discovered, reworked, or scrapped.	Quality is designed and built into the product. A nonconformance is a means for resolving the problems permanently.
A quality-control organization as a separate department inspects the output of manufacturing and evaluates the quality of production.	Quality is everyone's job. Total quality control includes all functions and individuals and all stages of manufacturing.
Quality is secondary to profits. To maximize profits, the sum of prevention, inspection, and failure costs is minimized.	Initial investment in quality is key to long-term profits. The book value of nonconformances is not simply deducted from profits.
Catch mistakes and fix them. Units are routed to manufacturing and inspection several times to pass inspection.	Do it right the first time. Quality at the source is the key. Do not make mistakes. Quality is free if produced the first time.
Suppliers are adversaries and thus suspect. All products must have at least a second source. Order as needed and expedite.	Suppliers are trusted members of our team. Work with a primary source to ensure reliability and quality.
Buy from the lowest bidder. Competition among the suppliers will reduce the total cost.	Buy for quality and reliability. Information and profits may be shared with suppliers.

(continued)

Table 1-2. *(continued)*

Old image	New image
Quality is a function of manufacturing. The products have high quality if they are manufactured properly.	High quality depends on all stages from design to shipping, and is reached only if all functions work properly together.
Errors will be caught by the inspectors. Keep the production line moving by keeping a safety stock.	Do not pass on nonconformances. Stop the line if there is a quality problem. A safety stock of work in progress is a waste.
Produce as many units as possible in the shortest possible time to increase efficiency and utilization.	Produce effectively only what is needed, and only when it is needed for the quality requirement of the internal or external customer.
Use specialized workers on operations to reduce the time needed for training. Produce units on an assembly line with highly specialized, single-operation-type workers. Do not rotate workers; rotations may reduce efficiency.	Train workers for diversified jobs and high flexibility. Promote cross-training and job-sharing among workers.
The quality department is responsible for quality. Problems need not be communicated to and from manufacturing.	Quality consciousness is the responsibility of everyone involved. Suggestions and discussions are particularly welcomed.
Management must discern quality problems and delegate responsibility for improvement. Employees should carry out the plans.	Management depends on employees to identify and solve problems. Management works closely with employees to resolve problems permanently.
The worker is responsible for most quality problems. He should be disciplined and trained to perform properly.	Management systems are the cause of most quality problems. Workers should be allowed to participate in management.
Statistics is an exotic tool for quality engineers. Control charts are used to highlight the problems.	Every employee should have an understanding of statistical quality control, which is used to highlight areas for improvement.
Additional inventory is maintained to keep workers utilized. The worker's idle time is a waste.	Inventory is a waste. The workers may spend their nonproduction time in other productive functions.
Large lots are produced to increase quality and to reduce production cost and average setup time.	Setup should be reduced to allow for lot sizes of one. Lower lot size means lower lead time, higher flexibility, and less rework.

Source: Sepehri (*33*), used with permission.

tively and systematically monitor and evaluate the quality and appropriateness of patient care, pursue opportunities to improve patient care, and resolve identified problems." When such a program is implemented in hospitals, it is seldom central to the management of the organization. In fact, it is more likely to be a committee function that is independent of the management function, often reporting directly to a medical board. Quality may be considered a technical issue, rather than a business strategy for establishing a competitive position in the marketplace. Controlling costs may be part of the motivation for the program, but the approach is to reduce utilization, rather than to reduce costs by improving quality and productivity.

The most comprehensive quality-assurance program for clinical laboratories is probably that described by Eilers (*34*). He describes the missions, goals, and activities of quality assurance programs in health care, and outlines the major components (see Table 1-3). The proceedings of a conference on "Quality Assurance in Health Care" (*35*) describe the components in great detail, as does a later book by Bruce (*36*). Although drawing from industrial approaches, this quality-assurance program still falls short of being a quality-management program: it does not demonstrate the "quality first" principle of industrial quality management.

In most clinical laboratories, quality-assurance practices are not even as broadly defined as in Eilers's recommendations. Quality-assurance practices tend towards "quality control." Quality control involves many different procedures, e.g., checking for proper labeling and identification of specimens, checking reagent lot numbers, monitoring the temperature of heating baths, measuring the concentration of known samples, and plotting the results on control charts. There is a strong history and practice of statistical quality control in laboratories; although this by itself is not sufficient for a quality-management program, it is an essential part of one.

Table 1-3. Eilers's Recommended Quality-Assurance Program

1. Design control: facility, staffing, and assays for mix of health-care problems
2. Raw material control: standards, control, reagents, instruments, glassware, samples, personnel
3. Process control: internal, to calibrate and control process; external, to monitor and refine proficiency
4. Output control: each result in medical significance format
5. Reliability control: assay utilization correlated with health-care needs
6. Verification control: inspection and accreditation; workload and man-hour record; cost analysis

Source: Eilers (*34*), used with permission.

How does quality management impact on the cost-effectiveness of quality control and analytical processes?

Clinical laboratories are facilities where the production processes are analytical processes, rather than assembly or manufacturing processes. The principles of quality management should be directly applicable. An understanding of quality and cost as they relate to a production process is essential in considering any question of the cost-effectiveness of quality control. Furthermore, statistical quality control provides a base upon which a quality-management program can be built. It is a tool for detecting problems (analytical errors), which should then be prevented from occurring in the future, thus leading to improved quality (fewer errors), higher productivity, and lower cost (less repeat work, fewer repeat requests), and ultimately improving the competitive position of the hospital.

Because all analysts use statistical quality control to evaluate whether their own work achieves the required quality, statistical control provides a vehicle for working with analysts for quality improvement. Each analyst is aware of quality, and, with support, can be encouraged to put efforts into identifying and solving problems. The ultimate objective is the permanent elimination of problems, so that quality and productivity are improved. That would lead to cost-effective analytical processes.

What is cost-effective quality control?

Cost-effective quality control means the use of control procedures that maximize both the quality and productivity of analytical processes. In our view of "cost-effectiveness," cost is related to productivity and effectiveness is related to quality. A cost-effective control procedure is one which achieves high productivity and high quality at the same time.

By defining "cost-effective" in terms of quality and productivity, it is possible to apply the concepts of industrial quality management to the technical management of analytical processes in clinical laboratories. In later chapters we will describe how the control procedure affects the quality and productivity achieved by the analytical process.

Summary

The principles of industrial quality management provide an essential background for understanding what quality and cost really mean, how cost-effectiveness can be defined in operational terms, and what cost-effective quality control is all about. The following are the important principles:

• Quality takes priority over production and cost. Achieving satisfactory quality is more important than getting the product out the door.

• Quality improvement begins with management. Management commitment, leadership, and active participation are required.

• Top management must give quality equal consideration with finance, marketing, etc.

• Quality is related to customer needs. Quality means satisfying the customer's needs.

• Quality is achieved by preventing problems, not by correcting problems after they occur. Quality requires careful and detailed planning of all activities of the organization.

• Cost is understood in broad terms to include the costs of prevention, appraisal, and failure. Failure-costs, the costs of not having adequate quality, show up internally in terms of scrap and rework, and externally in terms of customer complaints and service.

• Quality improvement leads to financial savings. The cost of unsatisfactory quality is high, money that is already being expended. Increases in productivity are possible by improving quality. With increases in productivity come lower costs of production.

• Extensive education and continuing in-service training are required for everyone in the organization, including the top managers.

• Quality improvement occurs only when specific problems in the process or system are identified and corrected on a permanent basis.

• Quality is everyone's job and requires teamwork. Project teams, quality-improvement teams, and quality circles are mechanisms for solving problems.

• Quality is a continually improving target. Quality improvement must be an ongoing process. The goal is perfection, nothing less, and is to be pursued relentlessly.

• Quality is a way of managing an organization. It is a way of life to be firmly ingrained in all of the operations of the organization.

On the basis of these principles, quality is understood to mean providing goods or services that conform to the needs of the users or customers. Cost, as understood in broad terms that include failure costs, depends on quality and productivity. Cost-effectiveness, then, is related to quality and productivity, and we define "cost-effective quality control" to mean the use of control procedures that maximize both the quality and the productivity of analytical processes.

References

1. Bean E. Cause of quality-control problems might be managers—not workers. New York: Wall Street Journal, 1985; April 10:29.

2. Deming WE. Quality, productivity, and competitive position. Cambridge,

MA: Massachusetts Institute of Technology, Center for Advanced Study, 1982:1.

3. Management's five deadly sins [videotape]. Lake Orion, MI: Britannica Films.

4. Tools for survival I: Models for success. Washington, DC: American Association for Clinical Chemistry, 1985.

5. Health care in the 1990's: trends and strategies. Chicago, IL: Arthur Andersen & Co., 1985.

6. Crosby PB. Quality is free. New York: American Home Library, 1979.

7. AMH/86 accreditation manual for hospitals. Chicago, IL: Joint Commission on Accreditation of Hospitals, 1985.

8. Op. cit. (ref. *6*):13.

9. Ibid.:15.

10. Juran JM. Upper management and quality, 4th ed. Wilton, CT: Juran Institute, Inc., 1983:B-1.

11. Glossary and tables for statistical quality control. Milwaukee, WI: American Society for Quality Control, 1983.

12. Freund RA. Definitions and basic quality concepts. J Qual Technol 1985;17:50–6.

13. Op. cit. (ref. *2*):12.

14. Manual for laboratory workload recording method, 1985 ed. Skokie, IL: College of American Pathologists, 1985.

15. Feigenbaum AV. Total quality control: the new business strategy for profitability, market growth, productivity, and competitive leadership. Workshop sponsored by American Society for Quality Control, State University of Iowa Section, Iowa City, IA, March 30, 1985.

16. Jenkins LM, Hunt MR, Carey RN, Westgard JO. Workload recording—a tool for increasing laboratory efficiency. Lab Med 1976;7(7):36–40.

17. Feigenbaum AV. Total quality control. Harvard Bus Rev 1956;34(6):93–101.

18. Golden J. Cost cutters must adopt a more holistic approach. Clin Chem News 1985(April):5.

19. Hospitals' program offers rebates. Wisconsin State Journal, 1985;April 24.

20. Crosby PB. Quality without tears. New York: McGraw Hill Book Co., 1984;85–6.

21. Op. cit. (ref. *6*):19.

22. The quality man [videotape]. Films Inc., Wilmette, IL.

23. Op. cit. (ref. *20*):75.

24. Gambino R. Quality control: can we achieve error-free work? Med Lab Observer, 1985(March);37–40.

25. Mead EF. Building a corporate quality culture: a test case. Qual Prog 1985(March);10–3.

26. Lammi RE. What commitment is/is not. Qual Prog 1985(July);10–1.

27. MacKinnon N. Launching a drive for quality excellence. Qual Prog 1985(May);46–50.

28. Young JA. Teamwork is more easily praised than practiced. Qual Prog 1985(August);30–4.

29. Dewar DL. Quality circles: answers to 100 frequently asked questions. Red Bluff, CA: Quality Circle Institute, 1979.
30. Juran JM. Upper management and quality. Workshop sponsored by American Society for Quality Control, Rockford, IL, May 18, 1985.
31. Quality service. Special issue of Qual Prog 1985(June).
32. Schoenberg RJ. Japanese manufacturing techniques, nine hidden lessons in simplicity. New York: The Free Press, 1982.
33. Sepehri M. Quality control circles: a vehicle for just-in-time implementation. Qual Prog 1985(July);21–4.
34. Eilers RJ. Quality assurance in health care: missions, goals, activities. Clin Chem 1975;21:1357–67.
35. Rand RN, Eilers RJ, Lawson NS, Broughton A, eds. Quality assurance in health care: a critical appraisal of clinical chemistry. Washington, DC: American Association for Clinical Chemistry, 1980.
36. Bruce AW. Basic quality assurance and quality control in the clinical laboratory. Boston: Little, Brown and Co., 1984.

Addendum: Review of Approaches to Quality Management in Industry

It is not our intent to provide a comprehensive review of quality management in industry, but it will be useful to identify some well-established programs that illustrate important concepts, practical guidelines for implementation, and aids for training and education. Deming, Juran, Feigenbaum, and Crosby are all well-known for their leadership in industry today.

Although these industrial leaders differ somewhat in their approaches, they have many more points in common than they have differences. They all have the same basic belief in the importance of quality management, but they have different approaches for implementing a program of quality management.

Deming's Quality, Productivity, and Competitive Position

In 1950, General Douglas MacArthur brought W. Edwards Deming to Japan to help reconstruct Japanese industry. Deming, a statistician who has worked in government, industry, and academia, had at one time worked with Walter Shewhart, the father of statistical quality control. During the Second World War, Deming applied statistical control methods to help American industry improve the quality of its defense products. Perhaps ironically, many of the skills that helped America in its wartime production are the same skills that allowed Japanese industry to compete in peacetime production.

Deming strongly states the position that the problems in American industry are the result of poor management. He is uncompromising in his indictment of past management styles. In his quality-improvement approach, he outlines 14 points of "management obligations"—management responsibilities, things management must do to achieve quality (Table 1-4). These 14 points are discussed in great detail in his books *Quality, Productivity, and Competitive Position* and *Out of the Crisis,* which are replete with examples from industry.

Table 1-4. Deming's Fourteen Points for Management

1. Create constancy of purpose toward improvement of product and service, with the aim to become competitive and to stay in business, and to provide jobs.
2. Adopt the new philosophy. We are in a new economic age. Western management must awaken to the challenge, must learn their responsibilities, and take on leadership for change.
3. Cease dependence on inspection to achieve quality. Eliminate the need for inspection on a mass basis by building quality into the product in the first place.
4. End the practice of awarding business on the basis of price tag. Instead, minimize total cost. Move toward a single supplier for any one item, on a long-term relationship of loyalty and trust.
5. Improve constantly and forever the system of production and service, to improve quality and productivity, and thus constantly decrease costs.
6. Institute training on the job.
7. Institute leadership (see point 12 . . .). The aim of supervision should be to help people and machines and gadgets to do a better job. Supervision of management is in need of overhaul, as well as supervision of production workers.
8. Drive out fear, so that everyone may work effectively for the company.
9. Break down barriers between departments. People in research, design, sales, and production must work as a team, to foresee problems of production and in use that may be encountered with the product or service.
10. Eliminate slogans, exhortations, and targets for the work force asking for zero defects and new levels of productivity. Such exhortations only create adversarial relationships, as the bulk of the causes of low quality and low productivity belong to the system and thus lie beyond the power of the work force.

11a. Eliminate work standards (quotas) on the factory floor. Substitute leadership.

b. Eliminate management by objective. Eliminate management by numbers, numerical goals. Substitute leadership.

12a. Remove barriers that rob the hourly worker of his right to pride of workmanship. The responsibility of supervisors must be changed from sheer numbers to quality.

b. Remove barriers that rob people in management and in engineering of their right to pride of workmanship. This means, *inter alia,* abolishment of the annual or merit rating and of management by objective. . . .

13. Institute a vigorous program of education and self-improvement.
14. Put everybody in the company to work to accomplish the transformation. The transformation is everybody's job.

Reprinted from *Out of the Crisis* by W. E. Deming by permission of MIT and W. E. Deming. Published by MIT, Center for Advanced Engineering Study, Cambridge, MA 02139.

The strength of Deming's approach is the use of statistical methods to aid decision making. This does not necessarily mean sophisticated statistical methods; simple methods of collecting and analyzing data such as histograms, graphs, control charts, etc. are often all that are necessary. The emphasis is on using data to help make the right decision, rather than making arbitrary decisions. Because of his emphasis on statistical methods, most statisticians involved in quality management have been influenced by Deming's approach.

Deming's approach is also widely appealing to workers because he is clearly concerned with the problems that limit their ability to do a good job. They understand that quality means jobs and it is their jobs that are of concern. He also states the problems very clearly to managers, in a way that gets their attention.

At age 85 (at the time of this writing), Deming continues to travel widely and lecture on "quality, productivity, and competitive position." Videotapes of his presentations are available, as is a documentary illustrating the application of the Deming approach in a Pontiac Fiero assembly plant. Many examples of the Deming approach are given in *Quality Progress,* a journal published by the American Society for Quality Control.

Juran on Quality Improvement

In the mid 1950s, Deming introduced J. M. Juran to Japanese industry to develop approaches for participative management. Deming had dealt with the top management of companies, and now the time had come for more widespread involvement of middle managers and workers. Whereas Deming stressed statistical methods, Juran focused on methods for making better use of people.

Juran, who has a varied career in industry, government, and academia, is a prolific writer. He has been involved in business management for many years and approaches managers with a good understanding of their problems. As president of The Juran Institute, he provides training courses and training materials on quality management to about 700 companies.

Juran stresses that quality is improved item by item, and occurs when a problem of quality is targeted for solution. In his terminology, a "quality improvement project" is a chronic problem scheduled for solution. Juran has developed many of the tools and approaches for managing quality-improvement projects. For example, the commonly used "Pareto diagram"—a histogram of number of errors (problems) arranged in order of most frequent to least frequent cause—was introduced by Juran and is widely used in identifying possible quality-improvement projects. The "Pareto principle," i.e., that a small number of causes are responsible for a high proportion of the problems, is the basis for selecting projects that have the potential to produce the most improvement. Projects are "legitimized" (officially approved for resources and support) by management, then solved by "project teams."

Juran is given much of the credit for the participative approach that resulted in "quality circles," but he carefully distinguishes "project teams" from "quality circles." Members of project teams are selected from management and workers, not just workers; participation is mandatory, not voluntary; the problems to be solved are interdepartmental, not departmental; and the duration of the team's existence is the time required to solve the problem (the teams are ad hoc, not continuous). The primary purpose of the project team is quality improvement, whereas the primary purpose of quality circles is human relations, with quality improvement as a secondary purpose.

In developing teams and teamwork, Juran extends the idea of "customer" or "user" to every individual in an organization. Each individual is at some time a customer (obtains materials and information from others in the organization), a processor (does something with those materials and information), and a producer (supplies the processed output to someone else).

Juran's ideas and contributions are so extensive that it is difficult to summarize them. He has contributed to almost all areas of quality management. The strength of his materials and approach is the focus on making quality improvements on a project-by-project basis. The Juran Institute provides a resource for companies who want training and assistance in implementing a quality-management program.

Feigenbaum's Total Quality Control

Armand V. Feigenbaum is an engineer who, in 1961, while a doctoral student at the Massachusetts Institute of Technology, first published his book on *Total Quality Control* (an expanded third edition was published in 1983). The Japanese system of "total quality control" has drawn considerably from this work. He was manager for worldwide manufacturing operations and quality control for General Electric Co. for 10 years, and now is president of General Systems Co., Inc., an international engineering firm that designs and installs quality-management systems.

Feigenbaum developed the concept of quality-costs (and its components of prevention-, appraisal-, and failure-costs) in the early 1950s. That concept is widely used by all industrial experts as a mechanism for getting management to understand the real cost of quality (or of lack of quality).

In a keynote address at the Conference on Quality Assurance in Health Care (*35*) sponsored by the American Association for Clinical

Chemistry, the College of American Pathologists, and the National Committee for Clinical Laboratory Standards, Feigenbaum defined "total quality control" to mean "the agreed, organization-wide, detailed operating work structure of technical, scientific, and managerial procedures for guiding the coordinated actions of the humans, the equipment and the information of the institution in the best and most practical ways, to assure user quality satisfaction and reasonable costs of quality." His broad program is outlined in Table 1-5.

The total quality-control program, a comprehensive approach that reflects a systems analysis of the whole organization, is described in detail in Feigenbaum's textbook, which is oriented toward professionals in the field of quality control and quality management.

Crosby's Quality Management

Philip B. Crosby is the author of two popular books on quality management: *Quality Is Free* and *Quality without Tears,* both of which can

Table 1-5. Feigenbaum's Total Quality-Control Program

1. Quality definition and evaluation, which deals with all the quality work related to the original specification and identification of what are intended quality requirements and standards.
2. Quality planning, which deals in an organized way with all the activities related to the establishment of how quality requirements are specificially to be evaluated.
3. Purchased material evaluation and control, which deals with the actions having to do with the control and assurance of all materials used.
4. Product control and evaluation, which includes the actual testing and analysis work and report determination.
5. Special process studies, which deal with the diagnosis of chronic quality deficiencies and with specific examinations to improve the level of quality.
6. Quality information feedback, which deals with the structured flow and cross-flow of data concerning quality.
7. Quality information equipment, which covers all the activities dealing with the testing, diagnostic, analysis, and data processing hardware, which are today so integral to quality activities.
8. Quality education, motivation, and training, which includes specific activities for improving quality skills, attitudes, and knowledge among all key individuals throughout the organization.
9. User quality evaluation, which deals with the continuing audit and quantification of the realities of user-oriented quality effectiveness.
10. Management of quality, which deals with the integration and assurance of satisfactory operation of these quality activities throughout the institution.

Source: Feigenbaum (*35*), used with permission.

be read easily by managers and workers. He has 34 years of experience in industry and was corporate vice-president of International Telephone and Telegraph Corp., responsible for worldwide quality operations. He is now chairman of Philip Crosby Associates, which consults with industry and provides training via its Quality College.

Crosby identifies four absolutes for quality management: (*a*) quality is the conformance to requirements; (*b*) the system of quality is prevention; (*c*) the performance standard is zero defects; and (*d*) the measurement of quality is the price of nonconformance.

He outlines a step-by-step quality-improvement program that provides a starting place for an organization wanting to implement a quality-management program (Table 1-6). Management commitment is

Table 1-6. Crosby's Quality Improvement Plan

1. Management commitment. Discuss the need for quality improvement with an emphasis on defect prevention. Prepare a quality policy for the organization.
2. Quality-improvement team. Form a team from the top managers of the different departments to guide the quality-improvement program and take the necessary actions.
3. Quality measurement. Determine the status of quality by documenting present performance.
4. Cost of quality evaluation. Estimate the quality-costs for the organization.
5. Quality awareness. Train managers to understand quality and quality improvement.
6. Corrective action. Solve initial problems identified through quality awareness training.
7. Establish an ad hoc committee for the zero defects program. Plan how to communicate to all employees the program for quality improvement and the goal of zero defects.
8. Supervisor training. Provide a formal orientation for supervisors before implementation of the plan.
9. Zero defects day. Present to all employees the organization's commitment to quality and the goal of zero defects.
10. Goal setting. Establish goals for improving present performance, as documented from earlier studies.
11. Error cause removal. Identify problems, solicit contributions from individuals concerning the causes, and implement solutions.
12. Recognition. Establish ways to provide recognition of individuals who contribute to improvements in quality.
13. Quality councils. Establish communications between personnel with special responsibilities for quality, particularly for those in different departments in the organization.
14. Do it over again.

Source: Crosby (6).

central and should be made evident by a written policy on quality. A quality-improvement team is organized to guide the quality-improvement program. The team develops measures of quality and estimates of the costs of quality. They organize in-service education and training to create an awareness of quality, leading to the involvement of all workers in the identification of problems and corrective actions. Ultimately, the emphasis is on prevention of problems: "doing the job right the first time."

Crosby provides guidelines for structuring in-service training programs. His Quality College offers courses to prepare personnel for training within their own organizations. Training materials are available, including several videotapes that are useful when introducing quality management in an organization.

Educational Materials for Quality Management

In developing an in-service training course in quality management, we have reviewed most of the following list of materials. Prices (as of 1985) are included to provide an estimate of the cost of different materials.

Journals

Quality Progress: monthly journal published by the American Society for Quality Control, 230 West Wells St., Milwaukee, WI 53203; yearly subscription, $21.00. A best buy for current applications in quality management.

Journal of Quality Technology: quarterly journal published by American Society for Quality Control; $11.00 for ASQC members, $21.00 for nonmembers. "The objective of the journal is to contribute to the technical advancement of the field of quality technology."

Books and Course Materials

Many of these books can be ordered through the American Society for Quality Control. See current issues of *Quality Progress* for book lists and order forms.

Crosby PB. Quality is free. New York: McGraw-Hill Book Co. 1979, 379 pp, $24.95; also published in paperback by American Home Library ($3.95) and available at popular bookstores.

Crosby PB. Quality without tears. New York: McGraw-Hill Book Co., 1984, 205 pp, $19.95; also available in paperback ($8.95) at popular bookstores.

Deming WE. Quality, productivity, and competitive position. Cambridge, MA: Massachusetts Institute of Technology, Center for Advanced Study, 1982, 392 pp, $45.00; course material for seminars that Dr. Deming conducts.

Deming WE. Out of the crisis. Cambridge, MA: Massachusetts Institute of Technology, Center for Advanced Study. June 1986, $49.00.

Feigenbaum AV. Total quality control, 3rd ed. New York: McGraw-Hill Book Co., 1983, 851 pp, $46.50; textbook.

Ishikawa K. Guide to quality control, 2nd ed. Tokyo: Asian Productivity Organization, 1982, 226 pp, $22.95; a good discussion of quality control and problem-solving techniques.

Ishikawa K (translated by DJ Lu). What is total quality control? The Japanese way. Englewood Cliffs, NJ: Prentice-Hall Inc., 1985, 205 pp, $22.95; a review of the history and current approaches to quality management in Japan.

Juran JM. Upper management and quality, 4th ed. Wilton, CT: Juran Institute, Inc., 1983, $55.00; course materials for workshops conducted by Dr. Juran.

Juran JM, Gryna FM Jr. Management of quality, 4th ed. Wilton, CT: Juran Institute, Inc., 1983, $80.00; course materials for workshops conducted by Dr. Juran and associates.

Juran JM, Gryna FM Jr, Bingham RS Jr, eds. Quality control handbook, 3rd ed. New York: McGraw-Hill Book Co., 1974, 1780 pp, $67.50; a reference manual.

Juran JM, Gryna FM Jr. Quality planning and analysis, 2nd ed. New York: McGraw-Hill Book Co., 1980, 629 pp, $46.95.

Juran JM. Managerial breakthrough, New York: McGraw-Hill Book Co., 1964, 396 pp, $34.95.

Videotapes

These tapes are listed in approximate order of usefulness. We have not reviewed the last four because they are expensive; however, they may be of interest to an organization making a commitment to widespread training.

The quality man. 1213 Wilmette Ave., Wilmette, IL 60091: Films Inc., 30 min, $495. A light and humorous introduction to Crosby's approach and philosophy, set as an interview by the British Broadcasting Co. while Crosby was on a golfing vacation in Scotland.

Roadmap for change—the Deming approach. 780 South Lapeer Rd., Lake Orion, MI 48035: Britannica Films, 30 min, $550. A documentary of the application of Deming's ideas in the Pontiac Fiero assembly plant, reviewing his 14 points and illustrating their application in a real situation; somewhat hard-hitting at management, but still suitable for an introductory training session.

In search of excellence. Films Inc., 90 min, $725. "Case studies" of

10 companies selected for excellence by Thomas J. Peters and Robert H. Waterman, Jr., for their book of the same name. Useful when integrated into a training program, it provides examples of some important aspects of quality management: the Leonard Grocery example is especially good for illustrating orientation to customers; the Disney example shows the importance of proper employee training; the Dana example shows employee involvement and participation in management; the North American Tool and Dye example illustrates management commitment to establish credibility with workers. Other examples may be useful in some settings, but are more oriented to other industries.

Management's five deadly diseases. Britannica Films, 15 min, $350. In an interview, Dr. Deming points out specific management problems and confronts management with serious issues; best used after some introduction and study of quality management.

Tools for survival I: Models for success; II: Optimizing productivity—human resources; III: Optimizing productivity—capital equipment acquisition. 1725 K St., N.W., Suite 1010, Washington, DC 20006: American Association for Clinical Chemistry, 30-min videotape in each course, $175 per course (including slides and workbook). These courses are directed specifically to clinical laboratories: course I presents the background for changing reimbursement for health-care organizations and suggests approaches for dealing with DRGs; course II contains many of the ideas on planning, organization, and teamwork as they apply to quality management, although the presentation puts priority on productivity; course III outlines methodology for analyzing the costs and benefits of new analytical processes (capital equipment).

The quality carol. Box 2369, Winter Park, FL 32790: Philip Crosby Associates, Inc., 45 min, $475. An introduction to quality management, showing a company learning about quality and its implications.

Why me? Philip Crosby Associates, $300. Presents situational problems for middle managers and illustrates "why" everyone must be concerned about doing it right the first time.

Zero defects: that's good enough. Philip Crosby Associates, 15 min, $275. Though dated by the dress of the characters, it may still be useful for presenting the concept of zero defects to workers.

Passion for excellence. Films Inc., 60 min, $795. A motivational presentation by Thomas J. Peters, based on his book of the same name; humorous and enjoyable, but not an organized presentation of the general principles of quality management.

A dramatic case study in quality and productivity. 77 Massachusetts Ave., Room 9-234, Cambridge, MA 02139: Massachusetts Institute of Technology Center for Advanced Engineering Study, three tapes, 35 min each, $500 each. Presents an example application of the Deming approach at Rogers Corporation; the total quality-control approach, initial training; manufacturing applications and staff-area applications; improving purchasing practices and supplier relationships; and developing better customer relations.

Transformation of American industry training system. Dayton, OH 45459: PQ Systems, 12 modules, $4125. "Transformation Seminars" also provided for instructors.

The Deming videotapes. Massachusetts Institute of Technology, 14 tapes, about 50 min each, $6300. Presentation by Dr. Deming of his course on quality, productivity, and competitive position.

Juran on quality improvement. 88 Danbury Rd., Wilton, CT 06897: Juran Institute, Inc., 16 tapes, $15 000. A complete presentation of Dr. Juran's course on quality improvement.

Workshops and Courses

See current issues of *Quality Progress* for announcements of many workshops and courses in quality control and quality management.

"Management of quality," FM Gryna, Jr, and RE Hoogstoel; Juran Institute, Inc., four days, $1200. Presented approximately monthly at various locations around the country; for schedule, phone 203-834-1700.

"Upper management and quality," JM Juran; Juran Institute, Inc., one day, $495. Presented approximately monthly at various locations around the country; generally coordinated with four-day course above.

"Quality improvement for services," AC Endres, JM Juran, and FM Gryna, Jr; Juran Institute, Inc., two days, $795. Presented quarterly at various locations around the country.

"Executive college," Philip Crosby Associates, Inc., two and one-half days, $1650. Presented at Crosby's Quality College in Winter Park, FL; regularly scheduled, phone 305-645-1733.

"Management college," Philip Crosby Associates, Inc., four and one-half days, $1800. Presented at Crosby's Quality College.

CHAPTER 2

Analytical Processes—The Production Processes in Clinical Laboratories

Managing quality requires an understanding of the systems or processes involved in producing the goods or services. Improvements in quality depend on changing a process to eliminate the causes of problems. The goal is to make it right or do it right the first time, thereby achieving the required quality while simultaneously improving productivity and reducing cost. To attain this goal, both managers and workers need to understand the production processes they use.

In clinical laboratories, the production processes are analytical processes. The products are test results. Patients' samples are analyzed by measuring some characteristic of a sample, often a chemical change caused by reacting the sought-for analyte with certain chemical reagents. The measurements are monitored by statistical quality-control procedures to assure their validity.

In this chapter, we review how analytical processes are established in clinical laboratories, identify critical characteristics of measurement procedures, and describe how statistical control procedures work. In reviewing some basic concepts and terminology regarding analytical processes, we will introduce terms and definitions recommended by professional organizations such as the International Federation of Clinical Chemistry (IFCC), the National Committee for Clinical Laboratory Standards (NCCLS), and the American Society for Quality Control (ASQC).

Analytical Processes

We use the term *analytical process* to refer to the protocols, materials, and equipment required to produce a reportable analytical result. An analytical process has two major parts, a measurement procedure and a control procedure. "Measurement procedure" refers to the analytical method proper, i.e., the reagents, the instrument, and the step-by-step directions for producing an analytical result. "Control procedure" refers to that part of the process concerned with testing the validity of the analytical result to determine whether it is reliable and can be reported.

Eisenhart (*1*) refers to "analytical process" by the term "measurement process," which he defines as "the realization of a method of measurement in terms of a particular apparatus, equipment, conditions, etc., that at best only approximate those prescribed. . . ." Those prescribed conditions are given in the "method of measurement," which defines the "specifications of the apparatus and equipment to be used, the operations to be performed, the conditions in which they are carried out. . . ." In defining these two terms, Eisenhart points out that principles may differ from practice: one method of measurement may lead to several different implementations, owing to the modifications that may be necessary in individual laboratories. An analytical process is a specific implementation of a certain measurement principle in an individual laboratory.

In clinical laboratories, the term commonly used to refer to the analytical process is *analytical method,* which is defined by the IFCC (*2*) as the "set of written instructions which describe the procedures, materials, and equipment, which are necessary for the analyst to obtain a result." Whether or not the instructions for statistical quality control are included as part of the "analytical method" depends on the interpretation of "result." Is the "result" the measurement made before its validity is assessed via statistical quality control, or is it the reportable "result" obtained after assessing the validity of the measurement?

To clearly distinguish the measurement part from the control part of the analytical process, we define *measurement procedure* as the protocol, materials, and equipment that are necessary for an analyst to obtain a measurement on a patient's sample. We define *control procedure* as the protocol and materials that are necessary for an analyst to assess the validity of a measurement on a patient's sample and thus whether a test result can be reported.

Establishing an Analytical Process

Figure 2-1 illustrates the many steps required to establish an analytical process in a clinical laboratory. Most analysts experience only a few of the steps. For example, an analyst may be involved in the routine operation of an analytical process without ever knowing the work that went into selecting and evaluating the process. Another analyst may be involved in evaluating new measurement procedures, and another may be concerned with assessing what kind of quality-control procedure should be used. Few analysts see an analytical process develop from beginning to end.

(*a*) *Determine medical needs.* The starting point is often a request by a physician for assistance in diagnosing a particular medical problem or monitoring a particular medical condition. The request may be a

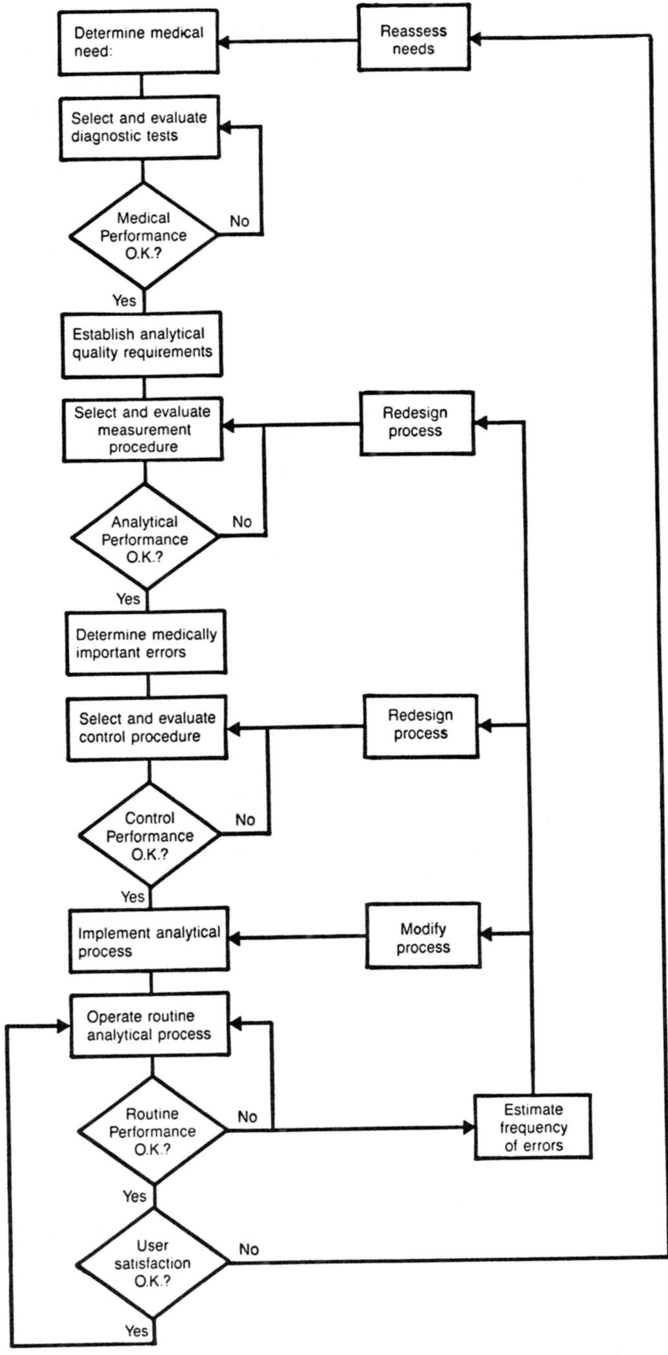

Fig. 2-1. Step-by-step procedures for establishing an analytical process

statement of a diagnostic problem with no identification of an analyte to be measured, but more often the physician already has some information about what analyte will provide medically useful information. Studies in the medical literature may describe how certain analytes correlate with a diagnostic situation or with changes in a medical condition, and several different tests may have been reported to satisfy the medical needs.

(*b*) *Select and evaluate the diagnostic test.* On the basis of studies in the literature, clinical experience, and recommendations of medical authorities, a diagnostic test is selected and documentation is sought to support the medical usefulness of the test. Quantitative assessments from clinical studies establish the diagnostic sensitivity and diagnostic specificity of the test (*3*). Clinical studies should be performed when the necessary information is unavailable from other sources.

(*c*) *Assess medical performance.* The predictive value and efficiency of the test can be calculated for the prevalence of disease in the population of interest (*3*). If the test results would provide useful information for the intended application, then a routine measurement procedure is sought. If the test results would not be medically useful, a different diagnostic test must be selected and evaluated.

(*d*) *Establish analytical requirements.* Once the medical usefulness of a test has been established, the analytical requirements must be defined. Both "application requirements"—factors such as specimen type, sample size, turnaround time, cost, etc.—and "performance requirements"—analytical range, analytical sensitivity and specificity, precision, and accuracy—must be defined (*4*). These requirements guide the selection and evaluation of the measurement procedure.

(*e*) *Select and evaluate a measurement procedure.* A measurement procedure is selected to satisfy the application requirements that have been defined. Experimental studies—analytical range, interference, recovery, replication, and comparison with another established measurement procedure—are conducted in the laboratory to test whether the measurement procedure satisfies the performance requirements (*4*).

(*f*) *Assess analytical performance.* The experimental results from method evaluation studies are analyzed statistically to provide estimates of analytical errors (*5*). The errors observed are compared with allowable limits of error (a total error specification) to judge the acceptability of analytical performance (*6*). If unacceptable, the measurement procedure is modified to improve its performance, or a new measurement procedure is selected, and the evaluation studies are repeated. If the analytical performance is acceptable, a quality-control procedure must be established before the measurement procedure can be implemented for routine operation.

(*g*) *Determine medically important errors.* When the measurement procedure is working properly, i.e., operating under conditions of stable performance, its errors are smaller than the allowable analytical error, as verified by the method evaluation studies. However, if the conditions for stable operation are altered, the size of the analytical errors may increase, perhaps invalidating the medical usefulness of the laboratory test. The size of these additional errors, "medically important errors," can be calculated from the total error specification and the errors observed in the method evaluation studies.

(*h*) *Select and evaluate a statistical control procedure.* A statistical control procedure is necessary to alert the analyst when medically important errors occur. The control procedure should be selected on the basis of the needed capabilities for error detection, as well as practical considerations related to its rate of false alarms, ease of use, training requirements, etc. The performance of the control procedure should be documented in quantitative terms, so that the chance of detecting the medically important errors is known.

(*i*) *Assess control performance.* The probability for detecting medically important errors is assessed to judge whether the control procedure is satisfactory for its intended purpose. One must also consider the probability for rejecting analytical runs that contain no errors (false alarms).

(*j*) *Implement the analytical process.* The analytical process, now a measurement procedure plus a control procedure, is implemented for routine operation. The operating protocol must be carefully documented and taught to laboratory personnel.

(*k*) *Operate the routine analytical process.* The process is scheduled for regular operation. Specimens are received, samples are prepared for analysis, tests are performed, and results are obtained.

(*l*) *Assess routine performance.* The routine operation of the process is monitored by use of the statistical control procedure. When analytical runs are judged to be "out of control," the results are discarded, the immediate problems are fixed, and the runs are repeated. When analytical runs are "in control," the results are reported.

(*m*) *Estimate the frequency of errors.* Recurring problems must be targeted for permanent removal. The frequency of errors should be documented to evaluate the seriousness of the problems, and the types of problems documented to help identify their causes. The analytical process should be modified to eliminate the causes permanently, or preventive maintenance procedures should be implemented to regularly remove the causes. With commitment to such problem-solving, the analytical process should, over time, become free of problems. As this occurs and the frequency of errors decreases, the demands on the statistical control procedure are reduced; consequently, the control procedure can be redesigned and simplified. If the frequency of errors cannot be reduced, one may have to change the process by selecting a new measurement procedure.

(*n*) *Assess user satisfaction.* As a stable, reliable analytical process develops, user satisfaction must be re-assessed. Medical needs may have changed in the time taken to establish the process. Test results may be interpreted more critically as a medical condition becomes better understood and as the usefulness of the test results becomes more apparent. New diagnostic and monitoring applications may have been found, completely changing the medical needs.

There are hundreds of diagnostic tests and analytical processes already established in clinical laboratories. Analysts will be involved more often in changing processes than in establishing processes from beginning to end. The analyst's role is usually to change from one measurement procedure to another as improved instrumentation becomes available. Although it would be easy to forget all of the other factors that are required for the test to be medically useful and to assume that a change in measurement procedure doesn't affect the clinical usefulness of the test or the requirements for quality control, the *diagnostic* sensitivity and specificity of a laboratory test can change with a change in measurement procedure, owing to differences in the *analytical* sensitivity and specificity of different measurement procedures. The analytical performance almost always changes when the measurement procedure is changed. Both of these changes affect the requirements for quality control and the appropriate design for cost-effective operation of the analytical process.

Quality, Analytical Quality

There are many quality requirements for laboratory tests (as described earlier in Table 1-1). Assuming that laboratory tests have been properly selected to provide medically useful information, then analytical quality becomes the basic requirement to be met if test results are to be useful in caring for patients. Providing the necessary analytical quality means conforming to the requirements of the user by limiting the sizes of the analytical errors that occur. An analytical error is any difference between an observed result and the correct or true value. Those errors or differences must be kept small so that they do not cause any misinterpretation or misuse of the test results.

Defects. According to the ASQC, a defect is "a departure of a quality characteristic from its intended level or state that occurs with a severity sufficient to cause an associated product or service not to satisfy intended normal, or reasonably foreseeable, usage requirements" (7). In clinical laboratories, defects are patients' results that have medically important errors.

Defect rate. The portion of test results having medically important errors is the defect rate for the analytical process. The defect rate will be a function of the frequency of medically important errors, the duration of those errors, and the capability of the control procedure to detect the errors; it may also depend on the type of analytical process. The defect rate provides a useful measure of the quality of an analytical process: the lower the defect rate, the higher the quality.

The number of defects can be limited by preventing their occurrence or by detecting them after they occur. The preferred approach for managing quality is prevention. Development of a stable (problem-free) measurement procedure provides the most cost-effective analytical process. When there are no errors occurring, there is no need for a detection procedure. Unfortunately, this ideal, stable operation is seldom achieved, and the performance of a measurement procedure generally must be monitored with a statistical quality-contol procedure.

Productivity, Process Utilization

There are many possible measures of productivity. Any ratio of "output" divided by "input" can be a measure of productivity; any units can be chosen. For describing the productivity of an analytical process, we are interested in the effective utilization of the process output. What portion of the measurements from an analytical process are correct and reportable patients' results; i.e., what is the test yield of an analytical process?

Test yield. Test yield can be estimated from the CAP Workload Recording Method (*8*) by dividing the number of patients' samples by the total number of samples: patients' samples, standards or calibrators, controls, repeat samples, and other miscellaneous samples (blanks, dilutions, etc.). This measure of productivity is affected by the type of analytical process, the number of calibrators and standards used, the number of controls analyzed, and the number of analytical runs discarded and repeated. A high test yield indicates effective utilization of process output, meaning high productivity for the analytical process.

Types of Analytical Processes

The quality and productivity of an analytical process depend, to some extent, on how calibrators, controls, and patients' samples are treated. It is sometimes assumed that any assay of a patient's sample would include recalibration of the procedure and simultaneous testing of control samples—a "batch" type of analytical process—but today's instrument systems are not necessarily operated this way. "Simultaneous batch" processes, for example, operate almost continuously, with test results being reported every 5 to 15 min; "random access" analyzers are calibrated very infrequently (at one- to three-month intervals), controlled periodically (daily, weekly), but can analyze patients' samples anytime, night or day.

Batch process. A group of patients' samples are assayed with calibrators and controls in an analytical run. All the samples are analyzed in sequence according to the order described in the protocol—usually calibrators first, followed by controls and patients' samples. The entire batch is processed as a group, experiencing the same step-by-step manipulations at the same time or in regular increments, one after another. Examples are manual methods, single-channel AutoAnalyzers, and centrifugal analyzers.

Simultaneous batch process. Calibrators, controls, and patients' samples are assayed in sequence for several different analytes at the same time. In effect, several batches are assayed simultaneously. An example is Technicon's SMAC analyzer (*S*imultaneous *M*ultichannel *A*nalysis with *C*omputer).

Random access process. Calibrators and controls are assayed periodically, at frequencies and intervals that depend on the stability of the measurement procedure. The control status of the measurement procedure is determined before the patients' samples are assayed. Once the process is verified to be in control, then the patients' samples are assayed individually or in small groups at any time until the next scheduled check for control status. An example is the Du Pont *A*utomatic *C*linical *A*nalyzer (*aca*).

The Measurement Procedure

Measurement procedures must be subject to careful development and evaluation by industry and by the clinical laboratory before statistical control procedures are applied. Industry provides most of the reagents and analytical instruments, and therefore assumes much of the responsibility for the development of measurement procedures. Clinical laboratories are responsible for performing method-evaluation studies and determining whether a measurement procedure is acceptable for their needs.

These efforts should identify and eliminate *assignable causes,* i.e., factors that contribute to variation and that are feasible to identify and eliminate (7). Many analytical errors can be discovered and their causes removed by careful choice and optimization of the conditions for the measurement procedure. The elimination of such errors provides an operating condition known as a *state of statistical control,* where only chance or random causes affect the measurement procedure (7). Unless such developmental efforts are carried out, a measurement procedure will be difficult to control under routine laboratory operation.

The resulting stable measurement procedure must attain the performance necessary for the analytical results to be medically useful. There is little value in applying statistical quality control if a measurement procedure does not provide medically useful results under stable operation.

Performance Characteristics

The performance of a measurement procedure is generally described in terms of precision and accuracy, but the frequency and duration of analytical errors are also important for assessing its stability of operation.

Precision. The IFCC (2) defines precision as "the agreement between replicate measurements. It has no numerical value." Precision reflects the ability of a measurement procedure to produce the same result again and again. The term *imprecision* is often used to describe the disagreement between the replicate measurements; it is defined by the IFCC as the "standard deviation or coefficient of variation of the results of a set of replicate measurements."

The distribution of measurements is generally described by a gaussian or "normal" curve, whose width is a function of the magnitude of the standard deviation. Figure 2-2 shows a gaussian distribution of measurements both above and below the mean ($\bar{x}$). The percentage of measurements that are expected to fall within certain limits (multiples of the standard deviation) of the mean, s, is as follows: 68.2% within ±1.0s, 90.0% within ±1.65s, 95.0% within ±1.96s, 95.5% within ±2.0s, 99.0% within ±2.58s, and 99.7% within ±3.0s.

Inherent imprecision. Every measurement procedure is subject to a certain amount of imprecision. None produces exactly the same result again and again, even when operating under optimal conditions. We use the term inherent imprecision to refer to the standard deviation or coefficient of variation of the results in a set of replicate measurements when the measurement procedure is operating under stable conditions.

Accuracy. The IFCC (2) defines accuracy as the "agreement between the best estimate of a quantity and its true value. It has no numerical value." Accuracy reflects the ability of the measurement procedure to give the correct result. The term *inaccuracy,* often used to describe the disagreement between the measured value and the true value, is defined by the IFCC as the "numerical difference between the mean of a set of replicate measurements and the true value." These IFCC definitions imply a "systematic error concept of accuracy"; i.e., only systematic differences are included when the mean of a group of replicates is used to estimate inaccuracy. We prefer to consider an "overall error concept of accuracy": that is, inaccuracy is the numerical differ-

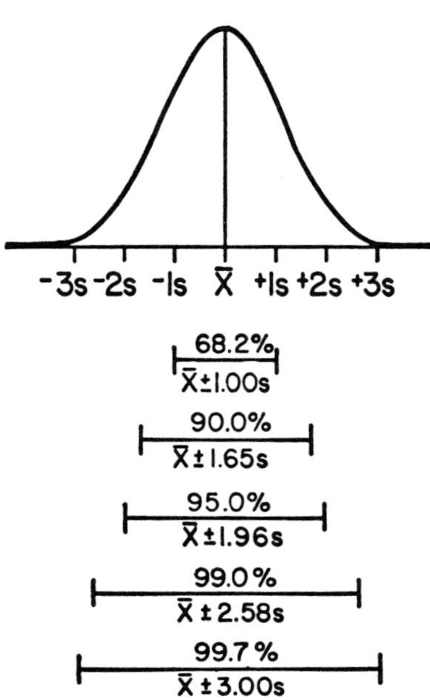

Fig. 2-2. Gaussian distribution, showing the percentage of total observations found within chosen limits about the mean

ence between a test result and the true value, and may include both random and systematic components of error (*9*).

Random error, systematic error, total error. In general, we will discuss imprecision and inaccuracy in terms of random and systematic errors, and will use total error to indicate our adoption of the "overall error concept of accuracy." The use of this terminology, we think, more clearly indicates the kinds of errors that are of concern. *Random error* is an error that can be either positive or negative, the direction and exact magnitude of which cannot be predicted, resulting in imprecision. *Systematic error* is an error that is always in one direction, resulting in inaccuracy. *Total error* is the net or combined effect of random and systematic errors.

Figure 2-3 illustrates the nature of these different types of errors. Replicate measurements of a single solution or specimen will produce a certain distribution, as shown by the observed values. The amount of random error, shown by the width of this distribution, can be expressed as a certain multiple of the standard deviation—in this case, ±2.58s limits, which include 99% of the measurements. Systematic error is shown by the difference between the mean of the distribution ($\bar{x}$) and the true value (μ). The total error is a sum of the random and systematic errors, assuming the "worst case" situation, where the

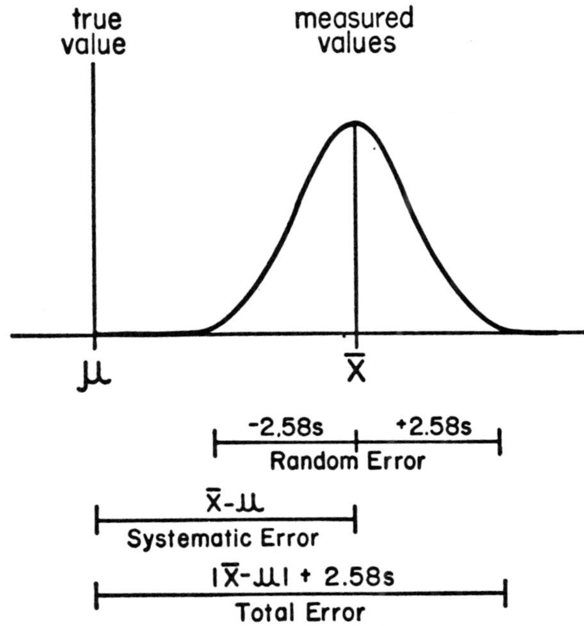

Fig. 2-3. Random error, systematic error, and total error defined

two errors have the same sign and add together to give a total error greater than either the random or systematic components. Because the random error can be either positive or negative, it potentially can always add to the systematic error to make the total error larger.

Frequency of errors. A stable measurement procedure would have no errors, except for its inherent imprecision or random error. The instability of a measurement procedure can be described by its frequency (of occurrence) of errors. However, information on the frequency of errors—the portion of samples (or runs) in which medically important errors occur—is difficult to obtain because it depends on the specific implementation and maintenance of a measurement procedure in an individual laboratory. Nonetheless, it is an important characteristic and should be considered when selecting or designing a control procedure.

Duration of errors. Not only the frequency but also the duration (length of occurrence) of errors is important. The quality and productivity of an analytical process depend on the number of runs in which medically important errors occur. That number is a function of the frequency of occurrence and the length of occurrence.

Intermittent errors are errors that occur in an individual run, but not necessarily in the subsequent runs; the errors are independent from one run to another, and do not persist. Persistent errors are errors that, once they occur, are present in the subsequent runs until detected and removed; the errors are not independent from one run to another. Persistent errors, because they last longer, are a more serious problem than intermittent errors.

Requirements for Analytical Quality

Analytical quality is concerned with the correctness of a test result, or its closeness to the true value. Feigenbaum (*10*) lists as the first point of his total quality-control program the need for "quality definition and evaluation, [which] deals with all the quality work related to the original specification and identification of what are intended quality requirements and standards" (see Table 1-5).

Quality specifications. Specifications for analytical quality that are useful for clinical analyses are the amount of analytical error that can be tolerated in the final test result without compromising its interpretation or medical usefulness in the care and treatment of the patient. Specifications for allowable analytical errors have been previously recommended for use when evaluating the performance of a measurement procedure in method evaluation studies (*9*). Those specifications can also be applied to the routine operation of an analytical process, for example, in the form of an allowable standard deviation (s_a, a precision specification), an allowable bias (b_a, an accuracy specification, systematic error concept), and an allowable total error (TE_a, an accuracy specification, overall error concept).

Figure 2-4 illustrates these different error specifications. Again, the distribution shown is of repeated measurements of a single solution. A precision specification describes the maximum width of the distribution. An accuracy specification describes the maximum difference between the mean of that distribution and the true value (μ) for a sample. A total error specification describes the maximum difference between the result of an individual measurement and the true value (μ).

Application in method evaluation. Criteria based on a total error specification can be used to judge whether the analytical performance of a measurement procedure is acceptable (*6*). Table 2-1 lists the types of errors, the experiments from which they can be estimated, and the criteria for judging their acceptability. These criteria allow a 1% defect rate; i.e., TE_a is defined as a 99% limit for errors, allowing only 1% of the samples to have errors greater than TE_a. A complete discussion of the formulation and derivation of these criteria is presented elsewhere (*4,6*), but the general nature of the criteria can be seen from the relationships in Figures 2-3 and 2-4. Note that we now recommend criteria that set a 1% defect rate (99% limits), rather than a 5% defect rate (95% limits) as in the earlier recommendations (*4,6*). The more

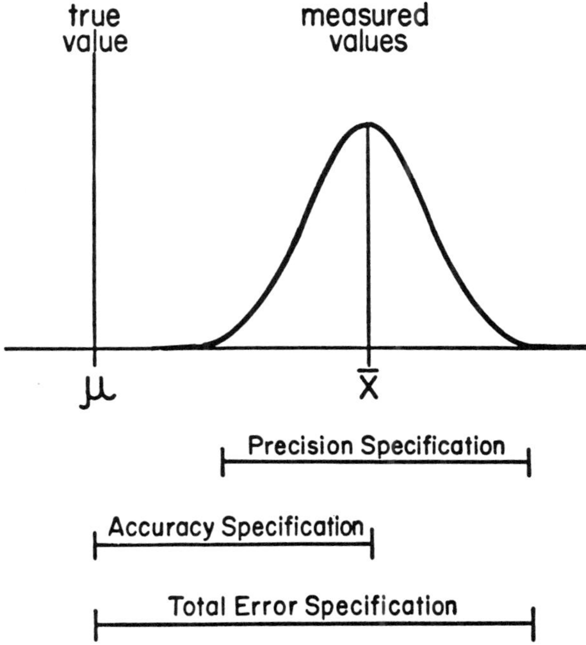

Fig. 2-4. The meaning of different specifications for analytical errors

Table 2-1. Criteria for Judging the Acceptability of the Precision and Accuracy of a Measurement Procedure by Method Evaluation Studies[a]

Error	How estimated	Criterion for acceptability
Random (RE)	Replication	$2.58s < TE_a$
Proportional (PE)	Recovery	$\|(\bar{R} - 100)(X_c/100)\| < TE_a$
Constant (CE)	Interference	$\|bias\| < TE_a$
Systematic (SE)	Comparison of methods	$\|(a + bX_c) - X_c\| < TE_a$
Total (TE)	Replication and comparison of methods	$2.58s + \|(a + bX_c) - X_c\| < TE_a$

[a] TE_a is the total error specification (a 99% limit, or a 1% defect rate for this set of criteria).
X_c is the medical decision level, or concentration of analyte where medical interpretation is critical.
$\bar{R}$ is the average recovery, in percent.
bias is the average difference from *t*-test calculations.
a is the *y*-intercept, from regression calculations.
b is the slope, from regression calculations.

demanding criteria are appropriate for assuring that the measurement procedure performs well within the required error limits when under stable operation.

Application in quality control. A total error specification can also be used to set the limits for errors occurring during the routine operation of an analytical process, as illustrated in Figure 2-5. The mean, assumed to represent the true value, is indicated by the central line perpendicular to the *x*-axis. The total error specification is indicated by the dashed lines at both sides of the distributions. Part *A* shows the error distribution for a measurement procedure under stable conditions. The quality

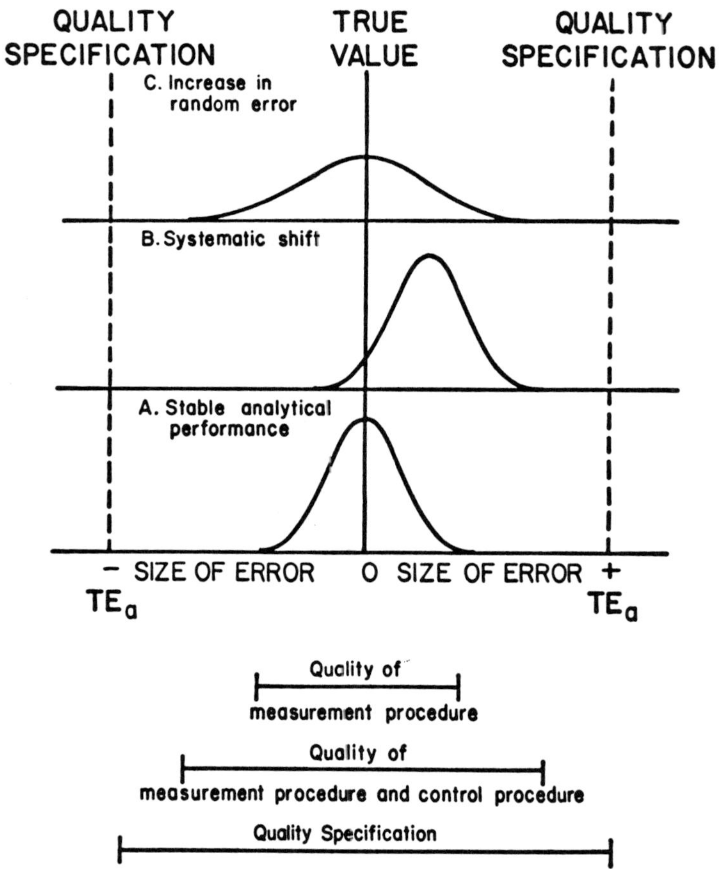

Fig. 2-5. Relationship between a total error specification and the quality of the measurement and control procedures

Reprinted with permission (*11*)

of the measurement procedure itself depends only on its inherent imprecision or inherent random error (if there is no bias during stable operation).

The quality of the analytical process, however, depends also on the performance of the control procedure. Part *B* illustrates an accuracy problem, in which a systematic error has caused the error distribution to be shifted from the previous mean. Part *C* shows a precision problem, in which the width of the error distribution has increased. The errors observed for the analytical process (measurement procedure plus control procedure) will be somewhat greater because the control procedure will have difficulty in detecting small systematic errors and small increases in random error. The sensitivity (error detection) of the control procedure is critical if random and systematic errors are to be detected before they become medically important.

Medically Important Errors

Medically important random errors are those increases in the standard deviation of the measurement procedure that cause the error distribution to exceed the total error specification (*11*). The *medically important systematic errors* are those shifts in the mean of the error distribution that cause the error distribution to exceed the total error specification (*11*).

The critical sizes of the medically important random and systematic errors are illustrated in Figure 2-6. If the critical sizes are defined as the errors that cause a *maximum* defect rate of 5%, as much as 5% of the tails of the error distribution can exceed TE_a. For random error, the problem is to calculate how much the standard deviation can increase before *both tails* of the distribution exceed the total error limits by the defined amount (here, 5%). For systematic error, the problem is to calculate how much the mean of the distribution can shift before *one tail* of the distribution exceeds the total error limit by the defined amount (5%).

Critical random error. For a 5% maximum defect rate (95% error limits), the critical random error (ΔRE_c) can be calculated as follows:

$$\Delta RE_c = s_a/s \qquad (2\text{-}1)$$

where s_a is the specified allowable standard deviation and s is the observed standard deviation of the measurement procedure. For the maximum defect rate of 5% specified here, TE_a is interpreted as a 95% limit, meaning that TE_a would be $1.96s_a$; therefore, $s_a = TE_a/1.96$. Substituting into equation 2-1 gives the following:

$$\Delta RE_c = TE_a/1.96s \qquad (2\text{-}2)$$

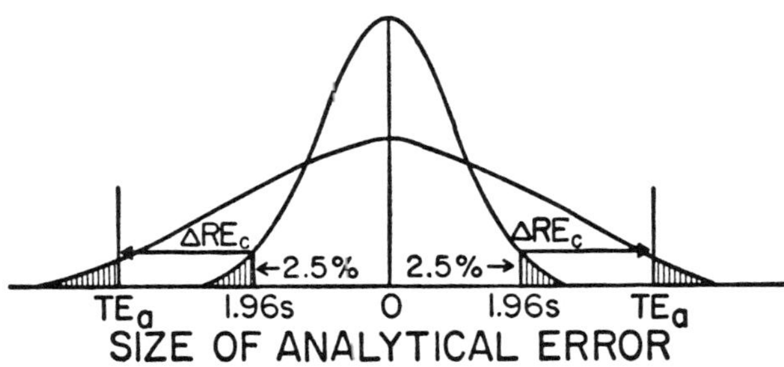

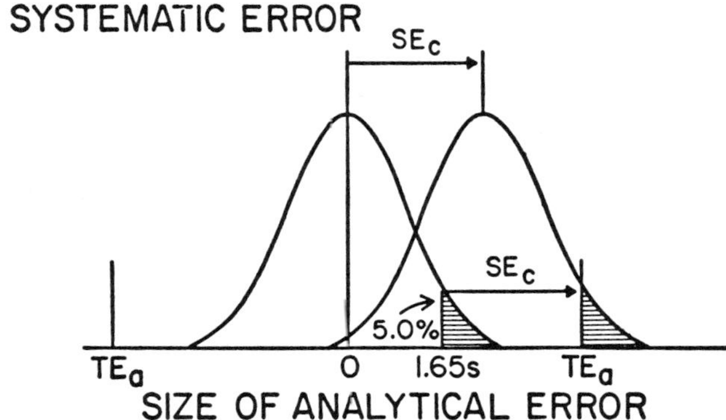

Fig. 2-6. Rationale for calculations of the sizes of medically important errors: critical random error and critical systematic error

Reprinted with permission (*23*)

The critical random error can be calculated either from s_a by equation 2-1 or from TE_a by equation 2-2 for a specified maximum defect rate of 5%. If a maximum defect rate of 1% is specified, then the 1.96 in the equation is replaced with 2.58. If a bias exists and the stable mean does not agree with the true value, then the bias must be subtracted from TE_a, as follows:

$$\Delta RE_c = (TE_a - \text{bias})/1.96s \tag{2-3}$$

Critical systematic error. For 5% of the area of one tail to exceed the total error specification, the mean must shift by 1.65s (see Figures 2-6 and 2-2; 90% confidence limits allow 5% in each tail of the distribution):

$$SE_c = TE_a - 1.65s \quad (2\text{-}4)$$

Dividing by s allows SE_c to be expressed as a multiple of s, rather than in concentration units:

$$SE_c/s = (TE_a - 1.65s)/s = (TE_a/s) - 1.65 \quad (2\text{-}5)$$

Defining SE_c/s as ΔSE_c gives the following equation:

$$\Delta SE_c = (TE_a/s) - 1.65 \quad (2\text{-}6)$$

The critical systematic error (ΔSE_c) can be calculated from TE_a by equation 2-6 when a maximum defect rate of 5% is specified. If the maximum defect rate is to be 1%, the 1.65 is replaced with 2.33. If a bias exists and the stable mean does not agree with the true value, then the amount of the bias should be subtracted from TE_a, as shown below:

$$\Delta SE_c = [(TE_a - \text{bias})/s] - 1.65 \quad (2\text{-}7)$$

Example calculations. Consider a measurement procedure for urea nitrogen. Ross (*12*) has recommended a medically allowable standard deviation (s_a) of 16 mg/L. If the observed monthly standard deviation (s) is 9 mg/L, what are the critical random and systematic errors that must be detectable by the control procedure?

The critical random error (ΔRE_c) can be calculated from equation 2-1 by dividing s_a by s: 16/9 = 1.78. The control procedure must be capable of detecting a 1.78-fold increase in the standard deviation of the method.

The critical systematic error (ΔSE_c) can be calculated from equation 2-6 once the specification has been expressed in terms of total error. For a maximum defect rate of 5%, 95% of the errors are to be included within the bounds of the error specification. The 95% limits for TE_a are therefore $1.96s_a$, or 31.4 mg/L. Dividing the allowable total error of 31.4 mg/L by the observed monthly standard deviation of 9 mg/L and subtracting 1.65 gives 1.83s for the critical systematic error. The control procedure must be able to detect a systematic shift equivalent to 1.83-fold the standard deviation of the method.

The Control Procedure

Managers and analysts need to understand how to monitor the quality of an analytical process during routine operation. Each analyst needs to understand how to judge the acceptance of an analytical run and how that judgment depends on the control procedure being used. Managers, in addition, should understand how the statistical control procedure can be selected or designed to optimize the quality and productivity of the analytical process.

Principles of Statistical Quality Control

The purpose of statistical quality control is to monitor a measurement procedure and alert the analyst when medically important errors have occurred. A direct way to check the quality of the laboratory product is to measure specimens with known concentrations (control solutions, control materials), then compare the observed results with the known values.

Control solutions, control materials. According to the IFCC, a control solution or control specimen is a "specimen or solution which is analyzed solely for quality control purposes, not for calibration" (2). We use the term control material or control product to mean a control solution that is available, often commercially, in liquid or lyophilized form and packaged in aliquots that can be prepared and used individually. Such materials are widely available for clinical chemistry analytes.

Control measurements, control observations. The analytical results obtained for control solutions (analyzed for purposes of quality control) are called control measurements or control observations. In many control procedures, the individual results are plotted and interpreted directly. Some procedures, however, require calculations to be performed on the control measurements before the data can be used to test control status. These derived or calculated values are called control statistics; for example, the mean of a group of six control measurements could be used as a control statistic.

Control procedures. Statistical techniques can be used to determine whether the control measurements are different from the known values. Such procedures are known as statistical quality-control procedures, or simply, quality-control procedures. Control procedures are commonly implemented by plotting control measurements (or statistics calculated from those measurements) on control charts; a control chart, therefore, is a statistical control procedure that provides a visual representation to aid interpretation.

Control charts. According to the ASQC, a control chart is "a graphical method for evaluating whether a process is or is not in a 'state of statistical control.' The determinations are made through a comparison of the values of some statistical measure(s) for an ordered series of samples, or subgroups, with control limits" (7).

Originally described for industrial applications by Shewhart (*13*) in the 1930s, control charts were introduced in clinical laboratories by

Levey and Jennings (*14*) in the early 1950s. Levey and Jennings described a control procedure based on the mean and range (difference) of duplicate measurements obtained for a single sample. Control charts, known as Levey–Jennings charts, have been commonly used in clinical laboratories since the 1960s. Actually, the charts embody the modifications described by Henry and Segalove (*15*): individual control values are plotted directly on a single chart to provide a simpler control procedure. Such individual-value control charts are the most commonly used control procedures in clinical laboratories today.

With the advent of computers (especially microcomputers) and commercially available quality-control software, other control techniques such as multi-rule charts (*16*) and cumulative sum charts (*17,18*) have become widely available. Many different kinds of control charts can be implemented, easily and practically, with the aid of computers.

By using control charts, analysts make decisions about the acceptability of the analytical results from individual analytical runs. Aliquots or samples of one or more stable control solution (control material, control product) are analyzed by the measurement procedure during each analytical run. The results are plotted on a control chart and compared with the control limits drawn on the chart; thus the analyst determines whether an analytical run is in control or out-of-control and whether the results for the patients' samples in that run are to be reported.

Control limits. According to the ASQC, control limits are the "limits on a control chart which are used as criteria for signaling the need for action, or for judging whether a set of data does or does not indicate a 'state of control' " (*7*). Control limits consist of upper and lower limits, which define a range of acceptable values. In general, an analytical run is judged to be in control when the control measurements fall within the control limits, and out of control when the control limits are exceeded.

Analytical run. According to the IFCC, an analytical run "usually refers to a set of consecutive assays performed without interruption. The results are usually calculated from the same set of calibration standard readings" (*2*). This definition does not easily apply to many of today's instrument systems, which are calibrated only daily, weekly, or even at monthly or longer intervals.

The NCCLS has offered a more applicable definition (*19*): "For purposes of quality control, an analytical run is an interval, that is, a period of time or series of measurements, within which the accuracy and precision of the measuring system is expected to be stable; between analytical runs, events may occur causing the measurement process to be susceptible to variations which are important to detect. The length of an analytical run must be defined appropriately for the specific analytical system and specific laboratory application. The manufacturer should recommend run length for the analytical system (MRRL) and the user should define run length for the specific application (UDRL)."

The NCCLS definition recognizes that the length of an analytical run depends on the stability of the measurement procedure and its susceptibility to errors. The manufacturer's recommended run length can be based on consideration of stability (a general characteristic of the instrument and reagent system when working properly), whereas the user-defined run length should be based on susceptibility considerations (specific characteristics related to the operating conditions in individual laboratories). The user's recommended run length should not exceed the manufacturer's recommended run length, but can be considerably shorter, depending on the operating conditions and needs of an individual laboratory.

What is most important for our purposes is to recognize that an analytical run, however defined, will include a certain number of patients' and control samples. An analytical run is that group of samples for which a decision is to be made concerning the validity of the measurements. The *number of control measurements per run, N,* is the actual number of control measurements available when judging the control status of the measurement procedure. N is critical for determining the performance characteristics of a control procedure.

Internal vs External Quality Control

Control samples may be submitted from sources outside the laboratory and the results returned to the sponsoring organization. When sponsored by professional organizations or manufacturers of instrument systems or control materials, such programs are commonly known as external quality control or external quality assessment. When submitted by regulatory organizations or when used for regulatory purposes, they are known as proficiency testing programs. Regardless of source, such programs provide for comparison of results between laboratories, and are also known as interlaboratory quality-control programs.

To integrate the operation of such programs with the intralaboratory or internal quality-control programs of individual laboratories, the same lot of control material is used daily in a group of laboratories. Manufacturers of control materials and professional organizations organize such programs and provide the data analysis and reporting services.

Interlaboratory programs provide a mechanism for assessing systematic errors by comparing the mean values from individual laboratories with the means for peer groups or with estimates of true values. The means for peer groups are calculated from the participants' results (with use of various criteria for selection or exclusion of results). In some situations, estimates of true values are available for test samples analyzed by definitive or reference-quality analytical processes (which are generally too expensive to be utilized in service laboratories). The difference between a laboratory's mean value and the program's estimate of the true value provides an estimate of systematic error. Additional judgments on the acceptability of performance can be made when a specification of the allowable analytical error is available.

Operation of a Levey–Jennings Control Procedure

Control measurements are obtained for the control samples assayed in an analytical run with the patients' samples. After performing whatever calculations and graphing are required for interpretation of the control data, the analyst decides whether the analytical run is acceptable. Results for the patients' samples are reported when the run is judged to be in control. When the run is judged to be out-of-control, the measurement procedure is investigated to determine whether a problem exists; if so, the problem is fixed, and the analytical run is repeated. Patients' results are generally not reported when an analytical run is considered out-of-control.

Records are kept of all control data, what decisions are made concerning whether runs are in or out-of-control, whether patients' results are reported, what analytical problems are encountered, and what actions remedied those problems. Control data are reviewed and summarized periodically (usually monthly), and control limits are updated (based on cumulative means and standard deviations).

Control materials. Most control procedures are based on the assay of stabilized samples, although it is possible to assay fresh samples from patients for control purposes. Stability is sometimes attained by freezing human serum, but more often by lyophilization, addition of stabilizing materials, or both. Suitable commercial materials are generally available and in use in most laboratories, although each material may have some limitations for certain analytes and certain instrument systems. One must select the control materials carefully, with specific attention to the different analytes to be tested; a single material may not be practical for all analytes.

In general, the most important properties are that the control materials behave like patients' samples, be stable throughout the periods of use, be available in sufficient quantity for a year or so of use, be appropriately apportioned for convenient use, and vary little from vial to vial. The source of materials—that is, human or animal—may be important for some analytes (e.g., enzymes).

The concentrations of analytes may be chosen to represent reference limits, appropriate medical-decision concentrations, or critical instrument-performance limits (such as the upper or lower limit of linearity). Often, two or three different concentrations of control materials should be assayed for each analyte. One can use sets of related materials (from a single manufacturer), which may provide additional information concerning the linearity of the measurement procedure, or the materials can be from different manufacturers, reducing the chance that they all will suffer from similar problems or limitations.

Data calculations. The measurement procedure that is to be controlled is first tested to characterize its analytical performance. Repeated measurements of control materials characterize the inherent imprecision or random error of the measurement procedure. The data are collected for a replication experiment, commonly over a 20-day period, with at least one control measurement per analytical run and one analytical run per day. Having two control measurements per run per day provides additional information about the within-run and between-run standard deviations, which may be advantageous in optimizing the performance of control procedures.

Mean, standard deviation, coefficient of variation. It is generally assumed that the distribution of these results or, more importantly, of the errors or differences between them is gaussian and can be described by the mean ($\bar{x}$) and standard deviation (s). The advantage of making this assumption is that one can then describe ranges of values that can be expected to include certain percentages of the measurements. Figure 2-2 shows a gaussian distribution and indicates the percentages of measurements expected to fall within ±1s, ±2s, and ±3s of the mean.

The mean and standard deviation can be calculated from the following equations:

$$\bar{x} = (\Sigma x_i)/n \qquad (2\text{-}8)$$

$$s = \sqrt{[n\Sigma x_i^2 - (\Sigma x_i)^2]/[n(n-1)]} \qquad (2\text{-}9)$$

where x_i is an individual control measurement and n is the total number of control measurements collected in the period being studied.

It is also common to describe precision by use of the coefficient of variation (CV), the relative standard deviation (the standard deviation expressed as a percentage of the mean):

$$CV = 100(s/\bar{x}) \qquad (2\text{-}10)$$

When n is only 20 or less, the estimates of the mean and standard deviation may not be reliable, and they should be revised when more control observations are accumulated. Additional data can be added to the data analysis by recording n, Σx_i, and $(\Sigma x_i)^2$. The cumulative totals for these terms, obtained by adding the values for the different data sets, are then used in equations 2-9 and 2-10 to estimate the mean and standard deviation for the cumulative data.

Table 2-2. Example Control Measurements for One Control Material during Five One-Month Periods[a]

Day	Month 1	Month 2	Month 3	Month 4	Month 5
1	98	100	97	101	100
2	97	109	98	100	96
3	95	102	102	99	101
4	103	104	92	100	102
5	100	97	104	96	104
6	104	105	100	100	100
7	92	98	95	98	96
8	94	100	100	97	101
9	102	96	104	103	99
10	95	103	101	107	105
11	100	97	101	104	100
12	93	97	99	96	95
13	100	96	97	104	101
14	106	97	112	105	99
15	112	104	92	101	90
16	94	99	105	102	98
17	96	105	105	102	106
18	97	94	101	102	100
19	103	95	95	101	101
20	104	97	100	104	97

[a] Simulated data, based on $\bar{x} = 100$, $s = 4.0$; **Source:** Westgard et al. (*76*).

Table 2-2 gives an example of simulated control data for five one-month periods, with 20 control observations per month. For the simulated data shown, the true mean was 100 and the true standard deviation was 4.0. The calculated monthly and cumulative means and standard deviations are summarized in Table 2-3. The first line for a month gives the mean and standard deviation for the control observations for that month, whereas the second line (shown in parentheses) gives the mean and standard deviation for the cumulative total of the control observations up through that month. The standard deviation changes more from month to month for the individual monthly data sets than for the cumulative data. Note that the accuracy of the estimates improves as the cumulative number of observations increases. The use of cumulative data should improve the reliability of the estimates of the mean and standard deviation, under the condition, of course, that the measurement procedure has remained stable (same $\bar{x}$ and s) over the period studied.

Table 2-3. Monthly (and Cumulative) Statistics—Means and Standard Deviations—Calculated from Control Data in Table 2-2

	Monthly totals			Calculated statistics	
Month	n	Σx_i	Σx_i^2	$\bar{x}$	s
1	20	1985	197 507	99.25	5.11
2	20 (40)	1995 (3980)	199 319 (396 825)	99.75 (99.50)	4.09 (4.46)
3	20 (60)	200 (5980)	200 434 (597 259)	100.00 (99.67)	4.78 (4.61)
4	20 (80)	2022 (9002)	204 592 (801 851)	101.10 (100.00)	2.97 (4.29)
5	20 (100)	1991 (9993)	198 457 (1 000 308)	99.55 (99.93)	3.65 (4.15)

Source: Westgard et al. (*76*).

Calculation of control limits. When the mean and standard deviation are known, one can predict the range of values that will be observed when the measurement procedure remains stable. Stable operation implies that there is no change in the accuracy and precision of the measurement procedure; therefore, the mean and the standard deviation remain constant. A shift in the mean or an increase in the standard deviation are due to additional analytical errors that do not represent the original stable operation. These are situations that the control procedure is supposed to detect.

Calculation of the range of values expected for the control material is based on the concept of confidence intervals. The mean is assumed to represent the true value for the control material, and the standard deviation is assumed to characterize the true gaussian distribution of the individual values. A range of acceptable values is then calculated as the mean ± some multiple of the standard deviation. Commonly, a 95% or 99% range of values is used to define acceptable performance, meaning that an analytical run is judged to be in control as long as the control observations fall within ±2s or ±3s (actually 95.45% and 99.73%, respectively; see Figure 2-2).

For the data in Tables 2-2 and 2-3, control limits ($\bar{x} \pm 2s$ and $\bar{x} \pm 3s$) are shown in Table 2-4. The control limits calculated from the cumulative data will be more reliable than those calculated from the individual monthly data sets, if the measurement procedure is indeed under stable operation.

Table 2-4. Control Limits Calculated for the Control Data in Table 2-2, with Use of the Means and Standard Deviations from Table 2-3

	Monthly (and cumulative) control limits	
Month	$\bar{x} \pm 2s$	$\bar{x} \pm 3s$
1	89.0–109.5	83.9–114.6
2	91.6–107.9 (90.6–108.4)	87.5–112.0 (86.1–112.9)
3	90.4–109.6 (90.4–108.9)	85.7–114.3 (85.8–113.5)
4	95.2–107.0 (91.4–108.6)	92.2–110.0 (87.1–112.9)
5	92.3–106.8 (91.6–108.2)	88.6–110.5 (87.5–112.4)

Source: Westgard et al. (*76*).

Preparation of control charts. The control observations are plotted on the *y*-axis vs time or run number on the *x*-axis. For a Levey–Jennings control chart, the *y*-axis is scaled to provide a concentration range of approximately $\bar{x} \pm 3s$ or $\pm 4s$. The *x*-axis is scaled to the period of interest, usually one month. Horizontal lines correspond to the mean and the control limits.

Figure 2-7 shows a Levey–Jennings control chart for which the control limits are set as $\bar{x} \pm 3s$ (as calculated from $\bar{x}$ of 100 and s of 4.0).

Interpretation of control data. Figure 2-8 shows how a Levey–Jennings chart looks when analytical problems occur. The first 10 data points show only the inherent imprecision of the measurement procedure. The middle 10 data points show an accuracy problem, or the effect of a systematic shift of the mean concentration. The last 10 data points show a precision problem, or an increase in the standard deviation of the measurement procedure.

The patterns of the control data reveal different kinds of analytical problems, and experienced analysts can generally recognize the analytical problems simply by viewing control charts. Less-experienced analysts may need more guidance in interpreting the control data, particularly if all analysts in the laboratory are expected to make the same interpretations from the same data. It is therefore necessary to define specific criteria for judging the control status of analytical runs.

A *control rule* is a decision criterion for interpreting control data and making a judgment on control status (*20*). To represent a control

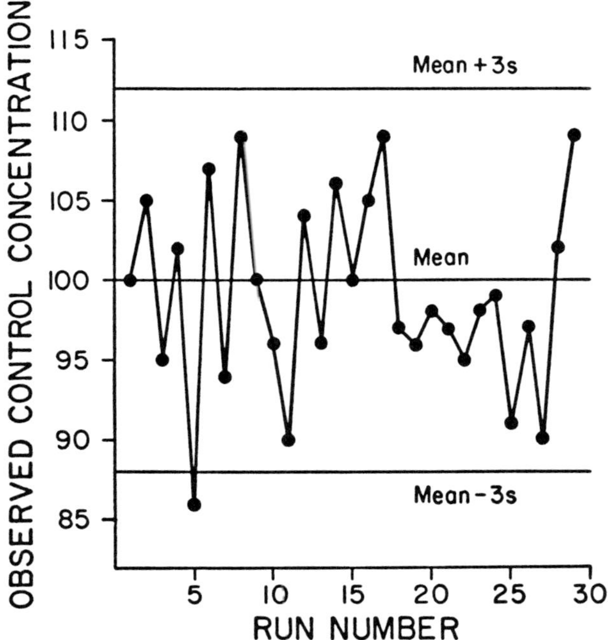

Fig. 2-7. Levey–Jennings quality-control chart: the observed measurements for a control procedure are plotted on the *y*-axis vs run number of the observations on the *x*-axis

Reprinted with permission (*23*)

rule, we use symbols of the form A_L, where A is the abbreviation for a particular statistic or is the number of control measurements, and L is the control limit. An analytical run is rejected when the control measurements fulfill the stated conditions, i.e., when a certain statistic or number of control measurements exceed the specified control limits. For example, 1_{2s} would symbolize the control rule that is implemented when a Levey–Jennings control chart has control limits set as $\bar{x} \pm 2s$, whereas 1_{3s} represents a Levey–Jennings control chart with control limits set as $\bar{x} \pm 3s$. In Chapter 3, we describe other control rules that can be used with "individual-value control charts"—control charts on which individual control measurements are plotted directly.

Other Quality-Control Charts

Other charts, such as the "cumulative sum chart," "mean chart," "standard deviation chart," and "range chart," may be used when the control measurements are subjected to prior calculations and the result-

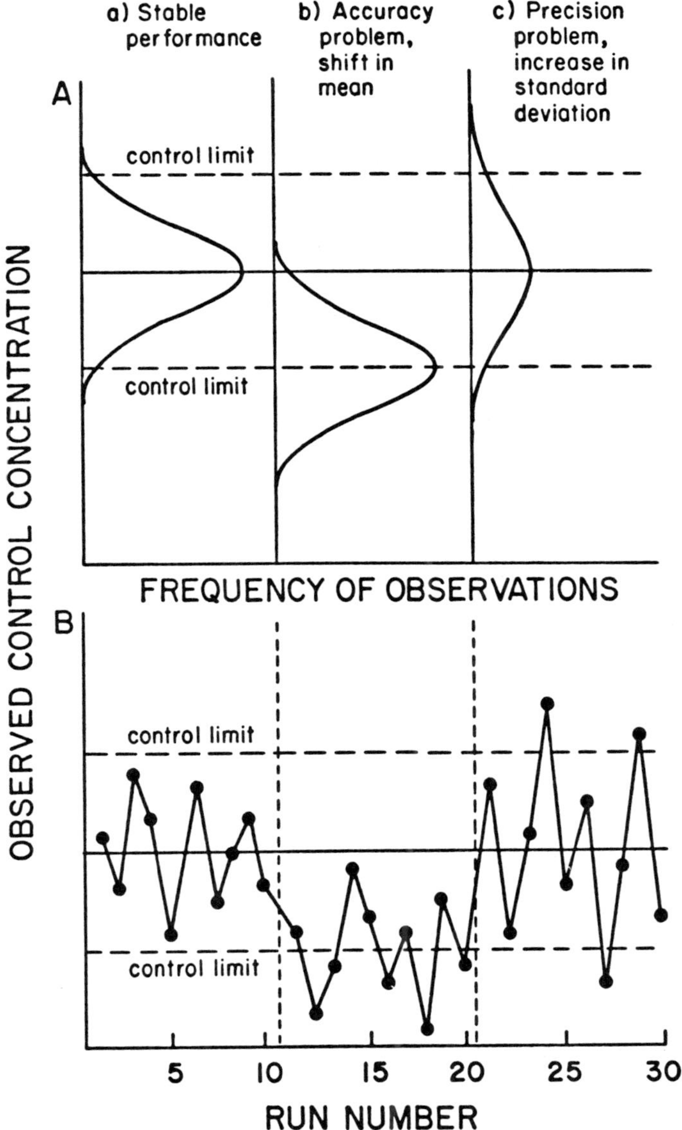

Fig. 2-8. Levey–Jennings quality-control chart, illustrating the effects of different types of analytical errors

Observations 1–10 represent results obtained during stable performance (affected only by the inherent imprecision or random error of the measurement procedure); observations 11–20 represent a systematic shift equivalent to the size of the standard deviation of the measurement procedure; and observations 21–30 represent an increase in random error caused by a doubling of the standard deviation of the measurement procedure. Reprinted with permission (*23*)

ing control statistics are plotted and interpreted. In most industrial applications these calculated values are charted, rather than the individual values of control measurements as done in clinical laboratories (*21*).

Cumulative sum control chart. Measurements on control materials are performed in the same manner as for a Levey–Jennings control procedure. For each control observation, its difference from a target value, usually the established mean of the control material, is calculated and added to the differences from previous control measurements to give the "cumulative sum." This "cusum" is plotted on the *y*-axis vs time or vs the number of the control observation (Figure 2-9). When control observations are scattered randomly about the mean of the control material, the plotted cusum will wander back and forth across the zero line of the cusum chart. When control observations are shifted to one side of the mean, the plotted cusum will steadily increase or decrease, moving farther and farther from the zero line of the chart.

Control status can be judged from the steepness or angle of the cusum line, qualitatively by visual estimation or quantitatively with the aid of "V-mask" templates—plastic overlays having a v-shaped cutout to establish the exact angle for the control limit (*17*). Alternatively, a numerical limit can be set for the cusum itself in a technique known as "decision limit" cusum (*18,22*). Examples of both techniques are given in Tietz's textbook (*23*).

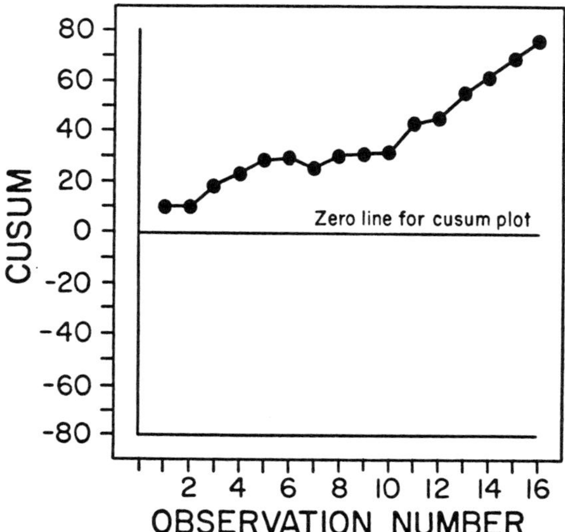

Fig. 2-9. Cumulative sum control chart

Reprinted with permission (*23*)

Mean, standard deviation, and range control charts. Shewhart, in his original work on quality-control charts (*13*), recommended obtaining several control measurements as a representative subgroup of a run, calculating the mean and standard deviation for that subgroup, and plotting them on an "x-bar chart" and a "S-chart," respectively, to monitor the accuracy and precision of a process. When N is less than 10, the standard

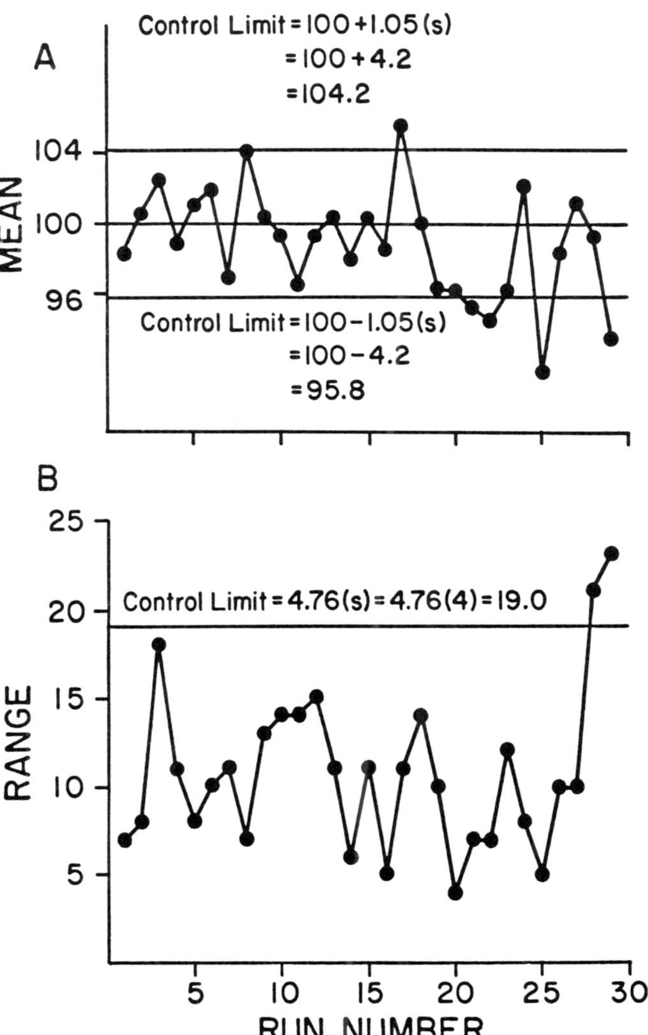

Fig. 2-10. Mean and range control charts

Reprinted with permission (*23*)

deviation is replaced by the range (the difference between the high and low values in the subgroup of N control measurements), which is plotted on an "R-chart" to monitor precision. Example mean and range charts are shown in Figure 2-10.

Control limits are calculated from the mean and standard deviation for the control material by using factors given in Table AI-2 in Appendix I. For the example in Figure 2-10 where N = 6, $\bar{x} = 100$, and s = 4, the control limits are chosen to allow a probability of 0.01 for false rejections, i.e., a 1% chance that a rejection signal could occur even though there are no analytical errors except for the inherent imprecision of the measurement procedure. The factor for calculating control limits for the mean is 1.05; the factor for calculating the *upper* control limit for the range is 4.76. A detailed discussion of mean and range charts is provided by Hainline (*24*).

Summary

An analytical process consists of a measurement procedure and a control procedure. Establishing an analytical process takes considerable time and effort, starting with developing a definition of medical needs and selecting a diagnostic test that provides medically useful information. If a routine measurement procedure is available, it must be evaluated to assure that its analytical performance is adequate to provide medically useful test results. A statistical quality-control procedure is selected for ongoing monitoring of performance. The resulting analytical process may be classified as a batch, simultaneous batch, or random access process, depending on how calibrators, controls, and patients' samples are analyzed.

The quality of an analytical process can be described by its defect rate, the portion of patients' results that have "medically important errors." The productivity of an analytical process can be described by its test yield, the portion of analytical measurements that are correct and reportable patients' results.

The critical characteristics of a measurement procedure are its precision and accuracy (characterizing stable operation), and the frequency and duration of errors (characterizing unstable operation). Analytical quality requirements should be specified to guide the selection and evaluation of the measurement procedure. On the basis of a total error specification and of the precision and accuracy observed in method-evaluation studies, one can calculate the magnitudes of "medically important errors," analytical errors large enough to compromise the medical usefulness of the results from laboratory tests.

The objective of the statistical quality-control procedure is to detect such errors. Statistical quality control can be performed by placing control solutions in routine analytical runs, measuring their concentrations, and comparing those concentrations with a range of acceptable values. A Levey–Jennings control chart is commonly used for plotting the control measurements and comparing them with acceptable values or control limits. Control limits are calculated from the mean and standard deviation determined for a particular control material. When control measurements exceed the control limits, an analytical run is judged to be out-of-control and patients' results obtained in the run are not reported.

Different kinds of control charts can be used, but the Levey–Jennings chart has been the most popular in clinical laboratories because it permits individual control measurements to be plotted directly, without the need for prior calculations. Other control charts, such as cusum charts and mean and range charts, although widely used in industry, have not been as common in clinical laboratories.

References

1. Eisenhart C. Realistic evaluation of the precision and accuracy of instrument calibration systems. J Res Natl Bur Stand Sect C 1963;67C:161–87.

2. Buttner J, Borth R, Boutwell JH, Broughton PMG. International Federation of Clinical Chemistry provisional recommendation on quality control in clinical chemistry. I. General principles and terminology. Clin Chem 1976;22:532–40.

3. Galen RS, Gambino SR. Beyond normality: the predictive value and efficiency of medical diagnoses. New York: John Wiley & Sons, 1975.

4. Westgard JO, de Vos DJ, Hunt MR, Quam EF, Carey RN, Garber CC. Method evaluation. Houston: Am Soc for Med Technol, 1978.

5. Westgard JO, Hunt MR. Use and interpretation of common statistical tests in method comparison studies. Clin Chem 1973;19:49–57.

6. Westgard JO, Carey RN, Wold S. Criteria for judging precision and accuracy in method development and evaluation. Clin Chem 1974;20:825–33.

7. Glossary and tables for statistical quality control. Milwaukee: Am Soc for Qual Control, 1983.

8. Manual for laboratory workload recording method, 1985 ed. Skokie, IL: College of American Pathologists, 1985.

9. Westgard JO. Precision and accuracy: concepts and assessment by method evaluation testing. Crit Rev Clin Lab Sci 1981;13:283–330.

10. Feigenbaum AV. What is total quality control? In: Rand RN, Eilers RJ, Lawson NS, Broughton A, eds. Quality assurance in health care: a critical appraisal of clinical chemistry. Washington, DC: Am Assoc for Clin Chem, 1980:3–12.

11. Westgard JO, Groth T, de Verdier C-H. Principles for developing improved quality control procedures. Scand J Clin Lab Invest 1984;44(suppl 172):19–41.

12. Ross JW. Precision performance standards: medical care and peer review criteria. Pathologist 1981;35:193–8.

13. Shewhart WA. Economic control of quality of the manufactured product. New York: Van Nostrand, 1983; reprint editions available from Am Soc for Qual Control, Milwaukee, WI.

14. Levey S, Jennings ER. The use of control charts in the clinical laboratory. Am J Clin Pathol 1950;20:1059–66.

15. Henry RJ, Segalove M. The running of standards in clinical chemistry and the use of the control chart. J Clin Pathol 1952;5:305–11.

16. Westgard JO, Barry PL, Hunt MR, Groth T. A multi-rule Shewhart chart for quality control in clinical chemistry. Clin Chem 1981;27:493–501.

17. Ewan WD. When and how to use cu-sum charts. Technometrics 1963;5:1–22.

18. Westgard JO, Groth T, Aronsson T, de Verdier C-H. Combined Shewhart-cusum control chart for improved quality control in clinical chemistry. Clin Chem 1977;23:1881–7.

19. Document C24-P. Internal quality control testing: principles and definitions; proposed guidelines. Villanova, PA: National Committee for Clinical Laboratory Standards, 1985.

20. Westgard JO, Groth T, Aronsson T, Falk H, de Verdier C-H. Performance characteristics for internal quality control: probabilities for false rejection and error detection. Clin Chem 1977;23:1857–67.

21. Duncan AJ. Quality control and industrial statistics, 4th ed. Homewood, IL: Richard D Irwin, Inc., 1974:431–84.

22. Davies OL, Goldsmith PL. Statistical methods in research and production, 4th ed. New York: Hafner Publishing Co., 1972:336–48.

23. Westgard JO, Klee GG. Quality assurance. In: Tietz NW, ed. Textbook of clinical chemistry. Philadelphia: WB Saunders Co., 1986:424–58.

24. Hainline A. Quality assurance: theoretical and practical aspects. In: Faulkner WR, Meites S, eds. Selected methods for the small clinical chemistry laboratory. Washington, DC: Am Assoc for Clin Chem, 1982:17–36.

CHAPTER 3

Characterizing the Quality of Statistical Control Procedures

Performing statistical quality control does not automatically assure that satisfactory quality is achieved. The size of the analytical errors that can be detected, and therefore the quality that can be assured, depend on the particular control procedure used. For example, analysts generally recognize that increasing the number of control measurements must have some effect on the quality assured, most likely improving the quality. Likewise, the use of different quality-control charts or different control rules for interpreting the control data must have some effect on quality, though it is difficult to predict what the effect will be.

How can the performance of a control procedure be evaluated? How can different control procedures be compared to determine which provides the best performance? To answer such questions, laboratory managers and analysts must understand the performance characteristics of statistical control procedures.

In this chapter, we describe an approach for characterizing the performance of control procedures quantitatively. With quantitative information, one can then evaluate and compare the performance of different control procedures, and, ultimately, select and design control procedures that detect medically important analytical errors.

Performance Characteristics of Statistical Control Procedures

A control procedure can give two kinds of signals: a signal to accept an analytical run, or a signal to reject an analytical run. A measurement procedure can provide two kinds of analytical runs: runs in which the patients' results are without errors, except for the inherent imprecision (or background random error), or runs in which the patients' results have errors in addition to the inherent imprecision.

Table 3-1 classifies the possible outcomes when a control procedure is applied to a measurement procedure. The "true reject" class (tr) includes the analytical runs with error for which the control procedure gives a reject signal. The "false reject" class (fr) includes the analytical

Table 3-1. Classification of Analytical Runs and Control Signals

Analytical run	Control signal: Reject	Control signal: Accept
With error	True reject (tr)	False accept (fa)
Without error	False reject (fr)	True accept (ta)

runs without error for which the control procedure gives a reject signal. The "false accept" (fa) class includes the analytical runs with error for which the control procedure gives an accept signal. The "true accept" class (ta) includes the analytical runs without error for which the control procedure gives an accept signal.

Probability for Rejection

Ideally, a control procedure should always give a reject signal when an analytical run yields results that have medically important errors. Otherwise, errors in the analytical results will be reported, reducing the quality of the analytical process. When an analytical run is without errors (except for the inherent imprecision), a control procedure should always give an accept signal, never a reject signal. Otherwise, the measurement procedure will be subjected to needless troubleshooting and repeat testing, reducing the productivity of the analytical process.

The chances for rejecting runs with errors and runs without errors can be described by probability terms that indicate the likelihood that the results of a given analytical run will be rejected. Probability can be thought of as the ratio of the number of actual occurrences of an event to the total number of possible occurrences, e.g., a ratio of the number of runs rejected to the total number of runs performed. As a ratio or proportion, a probability can never be less than zero or greater than one; thus, a probability is expressed by a number between 0.00 and 1.00, corresponding to "chances" from 0% to 100%.

The *probability for rejection, P,* is defined here as the probability that a control procedure will give a rejection signal for the results of an analytical run. A probability for rejection of 1.00 means that a rejection always occurs, whereas 0.00 means that a rejection never occurs. Two "probability-for-rejection" terms are needed to characterize the performance of a control procedure—one related to the number of true rejections, the other to the number of false rejections.

To develop quantitative performance characteristics, we express the number of runs in each class in Table 3-1 as follows. The number of analytical runs having erroneous results that are detected and correctly rejected (true rejects) would be given by n_{tr}; the number having errors that are not detected and therefore falsely accepted is n_{fa}; the number without errors that are falsely rejected is n_{fr}; the number without errors that are correctly accepted (true accepts) is n_{ta}. Using these terms, we can quantitatively describe the performance characteristics of a control procedure, as shown in Table 3-2. Two probability terms, the probability for error detection (P_{ed}) and the probability for false rejection (P_{fr}), can be described. The nature of these terms can be seen from their relationships to the different classes of analytical runs.

Probability for error detection. The probability for error detection is defined as the probability of rejecting an analytical run when its results contain errors in addition to the inherent imprecision of the measurement procedure (*1*). It is calculated as the number of runs with erroneous results that are rejected (n_{tr}) divided by the total number of runs with erroneous results ($n_{tr} + n_{fa}$). This term, P_{ed}, describes the portion of runs with error that are detected by the control procedure. Ideally, P_{ed} should be 1.00, meaning that there is a 100% chance of detecting a run with error.

Probability for false rejection. This is defined as the probability of rejecting an analytical run when there are no errors in its results, except for the inherent imprecision of the measurement procedure (*1*). This probability is calculated as the number of falsely rejected runs (n_{fr}) divided by the total number of runs without error ($n_{fr} + n_{ta}$). Symbolized by P_{fr}, this term describes the portion of runs without error that are rejected by the control procedure. Ideally, P_{fr} should be 0.00, meaning that there is a 0% chance of rejecting a run without error.

Table 3-2 provides a numerical example to clarify the two probability terms and their calculation. The probability for error detection is 100/

Table 3-2. Relationship of Performance Characteristics of a Control Procedure to the Numbers of Runs in Different Classes

	Control signal		
Analytical run	Reject	Accept	Totals
With error	n_{tr} (100)	n_{fa} (100)	$n_{tr} + n_{fa}$ (200)
Without error	n_{fr} (6)	n_{ta} (194)	$n_{fr} + n_{ta}$ (200)

Probability for error detection, $P_{ed} = n_{tr}/(n_{tr} + n_{fa}) = 100/200 = 0.50$

Probability for false rejection, $P_{fr} = n_{fr}/(n_{fr} + n_{ta}) = 6/200 = 0.03$

200 or 0.50, meaning that only half (50%) the runs that have errors are actually detected. The probability for false rejection is 6/200 or 0.03, meaning that three of every 100 runs (3%) would be rejected even though their results had no errors other than the inherent imprecision of the measurement procedure.

Descriptions of the performance characteristics of statistical control procedures in quality-control textbooks and journals generally use different terminology from that presented here. Instead of P_{ed}, the terms "probability for a β or type II error" or the "power" of the statistical test are used. For P_{fr}, the term "probability for an α or type I error" is used.

Determination of probabilities for rejection. Table 3-2 suggests that the performance characteristics can be determined by tabulating the number of runs in the different classes. However, performing an experimental study to do so is not practical because of the difficulties in documenting false rejects and false accepts. Too much time and effort would be required to investigate the actual results of the analytical runs to determine the correct classifications.

Fortunately, the performance characteristics of a control procedure can be determined from theory. A quality-control procedure is a statistical test, and its performance characteristics are statistical properties. For example, for a Levey–Jennings control chart with ±3s control limits and N = 1, the probabilities of rejecting errors of various sizes can be determined from the area of a gaussian curve that falls outside the 3s control limits (see Table AI-1 in Appendix I). When the only errors are those due to the inherent imprecision of the measurement procedure, the area outside each 3s control limit is 0.0013, for a total of 0.0026 or a false-rejection rate of 0.26%. When a systematic error causes the distribution to shift, one of the tails will exceed a 3s limit; for a 2.0s shift, the control limit cuts the tail at 1.0s, which contains 0.1587 of the area, meaning an error-detection rate of 15 to 16%. For $N > 1$ and for other kinds of control rules, the calculations become more complicated and are generally impractical for most laboratory analysts.

An alternative approach for obtaining this information is to do some experiments with numbers, to determine how a control procedure would respond to sets of control data having different types and magnitudes of errors. For example, given a set of control measurements obtained during stable operation, one can introduce an error condition by mathematically manipulating these values, then test the manipulated values to see whether an accept or reject signal is generated by the control procedure of interest. By doing this for many hundreds of sets of control data, one can use the proportion of rejected runs as an estimate of the probability for rejection.

To get complete information on the performance characteristics of a control procedure, we need to study three different error conditions: (*a*) no errors (except for the inherent imprecision), from which P_{fr} can be estimated; (*b*) a systematic shift in the mean ($\bar{x}$), from which P_{ed} can be estimated for a systematic error; and (*c*) an increase in the stable standard deviation (s), from which P_{ed} can be estimated for random error. In addition, the systematic and random errors may need to be studied at several different magnitudes to describe the general performance of a control procedure.

A practical way of doing these experiments with numbers is to use a computer to generate the numbers, introduce the errors, test the data, tabulate the results, and calculate the probability estimates. Such "computer simulation programs" attempt to simulate the conditions of interest in evaluating the performance of a control procedure. The simulation program permits the user to specify the mean and standard deviation for the measurement procedure, select the control procedure to be evaluated from a menu of procedures, and specify the number of control observations per run. Then the program performs the simulations to estimate the probabilities for rejection for a range of analytical errors and presents tabular and graphical summaries of the information (*2,3*). In addition, the program may be capable of taking into account such complicating factors as the relative sizes of the within- and between-run standard deviations, the effects of data rounding, and even the shape of the error distribution (deviations from gaussian behavior) (*4*).

Power-function graphs. One useful way to describe the performance of a control procedure is to plot the probability for rejection on the *y*-axis vs the size of error on the *x*-axis. The line obtained for each N (number of control measurements) is called a "power curve" because it describes the statistical "power" of the control procedure (its probability for rejection). "Power-function graphs," e.g., Figure 3-1, show the statistical power of the control procedure as a function of N and of the size of analytical error that is to be detected (*5*). The *y*-intercept gives the probability for false rejection because the analytical errors are at a minimum or zero, which is the condition of interest when considering false rejections. The probability for error detection is obtained by selecting on the *x*-axis the size of error that is of interest, drawing a vertical line to intersect the power curve, then reading across to the *y*-axis to determine the probability of detecting an error of that size.

Two power-function graphs are necessary, one for random error and one for systematic error. For random error, the *x*-axis is labeled ΔRE ("delta RE"), the size of random error to be detected, expressed as a factor by which the stable standard deviation of the measurement procedure has increased. For example, a ΔRE of 1.0 refers to the original stable standard deviation (s) of a measurement procedure; a ΔRE

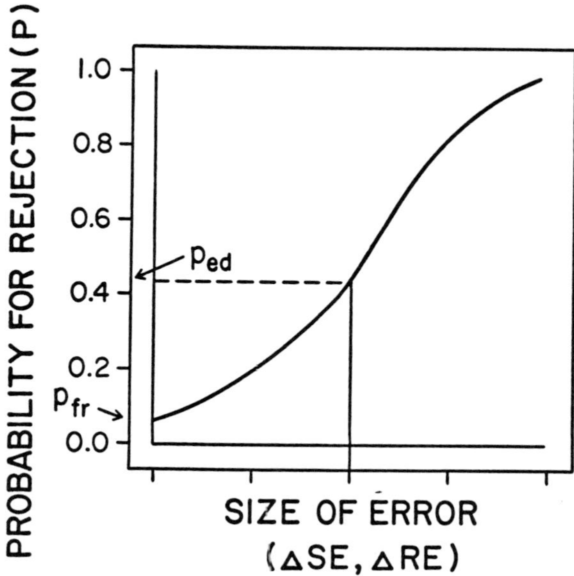

Fig. 3-1. Example of a power-function graph illustrating how to determine the probability for false rejection (P_{fr}) and the probability for error detection (P_{ed}); see text for details

of 1.5 indicates a 50% increase in s; a ΔRE of 2.0 indicates a 100% increase, or a doubling of s. For systematic error, the *x*-axis is labeled ΔSE, referring to the size of systematic error to be detected, given as a multiple of s. For example, a ΔSE of 1.0s indicates that the stable mean of the measurement procedure has shifted by an amount equal to s; a ΔSE of 2.0s indicates that the mean has shifted by an amount equal to two times s.

To illustrate with numerical examples, consider a urea nitrogen measurement procedure having $\bar{x}$ equal to 270 mg/L and s equal to 9 mg/L. A ΔRE of 1.5 would mean that s increases to 13.5 mg/L; a ΔRE of 2.0 would mean that s increases to 18 mg/L. A ΔSE of 1.0s would mean that $\bar{x}$ has shifted to either 279 mg/L or 261 mg/L; a ΔSE of 2.0s would mean that $\bar{x}$ has shifted to either 288 mg/L or 252 mg/L.

Figure 3-2 shows power-function graphs for a Levey–Jennings control chart having control limits set at ±2s. The graphs for random error and systematic error are illustrated. The different curves on the graphs represent different numbers of control observations per run (N). The probability for false rejection can be evaluated from either graph. P_{fr} increases with N, as shown by the increasing *y*-intercepts. For N = 1, P_{fr} is 0.05; for N = 2, P_{fr} is 0.10; and for N = 4, P_{fr} is 0.18. False

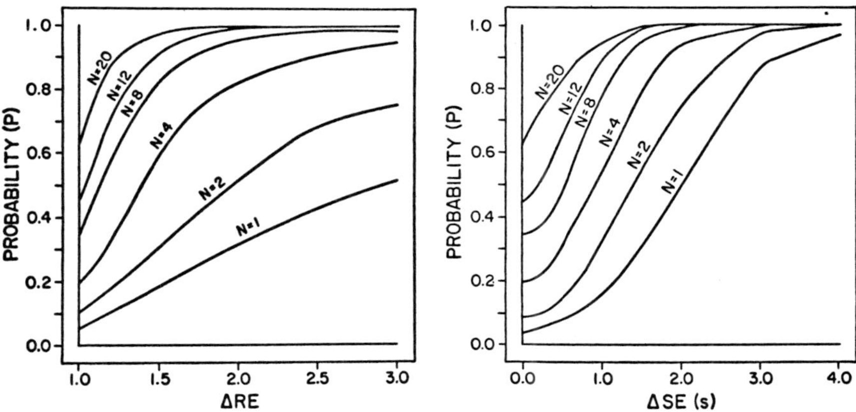

Fig. 3-2. Power-function graph for a Levey–Jennings control chart having ±2s control limits (1_{2s} control rule) for detecting random error (*left*) and systematic error (*right*)

The probability for rejection is plotted on the *y*-axis vs the size of the analytical error on the *x*-axis. For increases in random error (ΔRE), a value of 2.0 indicates a doubling of the original stable standard deviation (s) of the measurement procedure. For systematic error (ΔSE), a value of 2.0s indicates a systematic shift in the mean equivalent to twice the size of the original stable standard deviation of the measurement procedure. From Westgard and Groth (*5*), reprinted with permission

rejections are high whenever there are two or more control observations per run. Error detection appears to be high, but that is due in part to the increasing number of false rejections.

Figure 3-3 shows the power-function graphs when ±3s control limits are used on a Levey–Jennings chart. The probability for false rejection is very low, even when N increases to eight to 20 control observations per run. The probability for error detection is also quite low. For an increase in random error corresponding to a doubling of s, P_{ed} is 0.12 when N = 1, 0.20 when N = 2, and 0.42 when N = 4. For a systematic shift equivalent to 2.0s, P_{ed} is 0.15 when N = 1, 0.24 when N = 2, and 0.45 when N = 4.

In Appendix II, we provide power-function graphs for many of the control procedures in use in clinical laboratories. The probabilities for rejection were determined by computer simulation. The power curves are drawn point to point, which reveals the experimental uncertainty in the simulation studies; interpretation may occasionally require some visual averaging. We have provided graphs for $s_b = 0$, the ideal situation where the between-run standard deviation (s_b) is zero and the inherent imprecision is due only to the within-run standard deviation (s_w). Access to a computer simulation program would provide more comprehensive consideration of the effects of the within- and

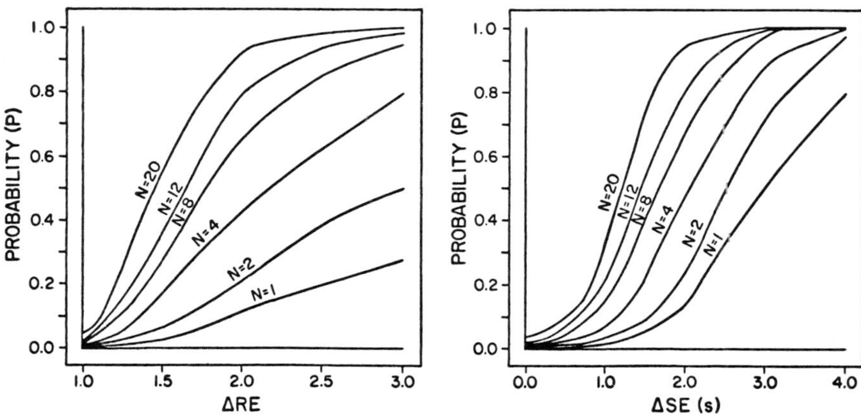

Fig. 3-3. Power-function graphs for a Levey–Jennings control chart having ±3s control limits (1_{3s} control rule) for detecting random error (*left*) and systematic error (*right*)

From Westgard and Groth (*5*), reprinted with permission

between-run standard deviations and also of the effects of data rounding.

Average Run Lengths

It may also be useful to describe the performance of a control procedure in terms of the average number of analytical runs that will occur before a run is rejected. This is called the "average run length" (ARL) and can be specified for both "acceptable quality" and "rejectable quality." The *average run length for acceptable quality* (ARL_a) refers to the situation where the only error present is the inherent imprecision of the measurement procedure. The *average run length for rejectable quality* (ARL_r) refers to the situation where errors are present, in addition to the inherent imprecision of the measurement procedure.

Persistent vs intermittent analytical errors. The ARL performance characteristics are important when the measurement procedure is subject to persistent analytical errors that continue (persist) from one run to the next until detected and removed. For intermittent errors—those that occur in an individual run, but not necessarily in the following runs—the probability terms (P_{ed}, P_{fr}) describe the chances of detecting the error and rejecting the analytical run. ARL calculations are not necessary for intermittent errors.

Calculation of average run lengths. For control procedures that depend only on the control measurements in the current run, the probability for rejection does not change from run to run, and the ARL can be calculated as shown by Duncan (*6*):

$$\text{ARL} = \frac{1}{P} \tag{3-1}$$

where P is the probability of rejection as determined for a single run in which the error occurs. ARL_a can be determined from $1/P_{fr}$ and ARL_r from $1/P_{ed}$.

For example, for the Levey–Jennings chart having 3s control limits and N = 4, P_{fr} is about 0.01 and the corresponding ARL_a is 100 (1/0.01 = 100). Thus, when the measurement procedure is operating under stable conditions, there will be an average of 100 runs between rejections. The lower the P_{fr} value, the greater the number of runs between rejections. For this same control procedure, P_{ed} is 0.45 for a 2s shift, and the corresponding ARL_r is 2.2 (1/0.45 = 2.2). That is, when an error occurs, it will take an average of 2.2 runs before the error is detected. The higher the P_{ed} value, the smaller the number of runs before the error condition is detected.

In addition to the average run length, the distribution of run lengths may be interesting. The distribution can be determined from a more general equation:

$$\text{ARL} = \sum_{r=1}^{\infty} r P_r Q_r \tag{3-2}$$

where r is the run number, P_r is the probability for rejection in the rth run, and Q_r is the proportion of runs with errors undetected up to the rth run.[1]

Table 3-3 illustrates the calculations for the case when P_{ed} is 0.45 and does not change from run to run. Column 1 gives the run number or run length; column 2 gives the probability for error detection in this run, as obtained from power-function graphs, assuming the error persists from the first run through this run; column 3 shows the proportion of the errors that are undetected prior to the given run (1 minus column 5 from the previous run); column 4 shows the proportion of

[1] Equation 3-2 is an equation for calculating the average of grouped data, the value for each group being r. The number of data in each group is the number of runs rejected, determined from the probability for rejection times the proportion of runs ($P_r \cdot Q_r$). The average is determined by multiplying the value of each group by the number in each group, then dividing by the total number, which is actually 1 because the number of runs is presented as a proportion. Thus, the summation of the products of the run length times the proportion of runs rejected at each run length gives the average run length (ARL).

Table 3-3. Example Calculation of Average Run Length (ARL) when the Probability for Error Detection (P_{ed}) Is Constant from Run to Run

		Proportion of errors			
Run no. (or run length)	P_{ed}, this run	Undetected before this run	Detected this run	Cumulative detected	Calculated contribution to ARL
1	0.450	1.000	0.450	0.450	0.450
2	0.450	0.550	0.248	0.698	0.495
3	0.450	0.303	0.136	0.834	0.408
4	0.450	0.166	0.075	0.908	0.299
5	0.450	0.092	0.041	0.950	0.206
6	0.450	0.050	0.023	0.972	0.136
7	0.450	0.028	0.012	0.985	0.087
8	0.450	0.015	0.007	0.992	0.055
9	0.450	0.008	0.004	0.995	0.034
10	0.450	0.005	0.002	0.997	0.021
11	0.450	0.003	0.001	0.999	0.013
12	0.450	0.001	0.001	0.999	0.008
13	0.450	0.001	0.000	1.000	0.004
14	0.450	0.001	0.000	1.000	0.003
15	0.450	0.000	0.000	1.000	0.002
16	0.450	0.000	0.000	1.000	0.001
17	0.450	0.000	0.000	1.000	0.001
18	0.450	0.000	0.000	1.000	0.000
19	0.450	0.000	0.000	1.000	0.000
20	0.450	0.000	0.000	1.000	0.000
				ARL =	2.222

errors detected in the given run (column 2 times column 3); column 5 shows the cumulative proportion of the errors detected up through the given run (sum of values in column 4 through this run); column 6 gives the contribution to the average run length (the run number in column 1 multiplied by the proportion of errors detected in the run in column 4); the summation of column 6 gives the average run length, which is 2.2 and agrees with the value calculated earlier from the simple formula $1/P$.

Figure 3-4 shows the distribution of run lengths (a plot of values in column 4 in Table 3-3 vs column 1). Although the average run length may be 2.2, it is obvious that as many as four or five runs will sometimes be accepted before an error is detected. From column 5 in Table 3-3 (the cumulative proportion of errors detected), 83% of

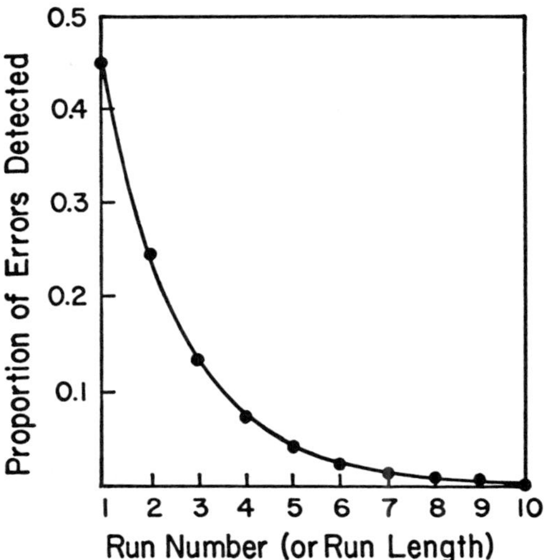

Fig. 3-4. For a Levey–Jennings control chart having ±3s control limits (1_{3s} control rule) with four control measurements (N = 4), distribution of run lengths for detecting a systematic shift (ΔSE) equivalent to 2.0s

the errors would be detected within the first three runs, leaving 17% to be detected after run lengths of four or more.

One can also use equation 3-2 to calculate the distribution of runs and the average run length when P changes from run to run. For control procedures that accumulate control measurements (cumulative sum procedures) or that include past or retrospective measurements (multi-rule procedures), P_{ed} increases from run to run when an error persists and goes undetected. The calculation of ARL_r cannot be made from the simple formula $1/P_{ed}$ because P_{ed} is not a constant. Chapter 4 includes some examples to illustrate these slightly more complicated situations.

The ARL calculations can easily be performed with electronic spreadsheets, such as Lotus 1-2-3 (Lotus Development Corp., Cambridge, MA 02142). A spreadsheet set up to handle 20 runs will usually suffice for calculating ARL for large errors. A spreadsheet for 100 runs may be necessary for smaller errors. Entry of the probabilities, calculation of all the terms, and printing of the worksheet takes only a minute or two for each estimation of ARL. See Appendix III for a description of a spreadsheet for performing these calculations.

Example Application: Urea Nitrogen

To illustrate how power functions and average run lengths can be used to evaluate and compare control procedures, consider the urea nitrogen example from Chapter 2. Recall that we calculated the critical sizes of medically important errors and found that ΔRE_c was equal to a 1.78-fold increase in s, and that ΔSE_c was equal to a shift in the mean equivalent to 1.83s. Now let us evaluate the use of Levey–Jennings control procedures for controlling the procedure for measuring urea nitrogen.

From the power-function graphs for the Levey–Jennings chart having ±3s control limits, we see that the probability for false rejection is 0.01 or less when N = 1 through 4. Therefore, ARL_a will be 100 (1/0.01 from equation 3-1). To determine the probabilities for detecting the critical random error, we draw a vertical line from 1.78 on the *x*-axis of the power-function graph for random error, as shown in Figure 3-5 (left), then read the probabilities from the *y*-axis. If a random error of that size occurs, there is only a 7% chance of detection when N = 1; 14% for N = 2; 33% for N = 4; and 51% for N = 8 (ARL_rs of 1/0.07 = 14, 1/0.14 = 7.1, 1/0.33 = 3.0, and 1/0.51 = 2.0, respectively). More than 20 control measurements would be required to have a 90% chance of detecting the critical random error.

To determine the probabilities for detecting the critical systematic error, we draw a vertical line from 1.83 on the *x*-axis of the power-function graph for systematic error, as shown in Figure 3-5 (right). If a systematic error of that size occurs, there is only a 10% chance of detection when N = 1; 17% when N = 2; 38% when N = 4; and 57% when N = 8 (ARL_rs of 1/0.10 = 10, 1/0.17 = 5.9, 1/0.38 = 2.6, and 1/0.58 = 1.7, respectively). Approximately 20 control measure-

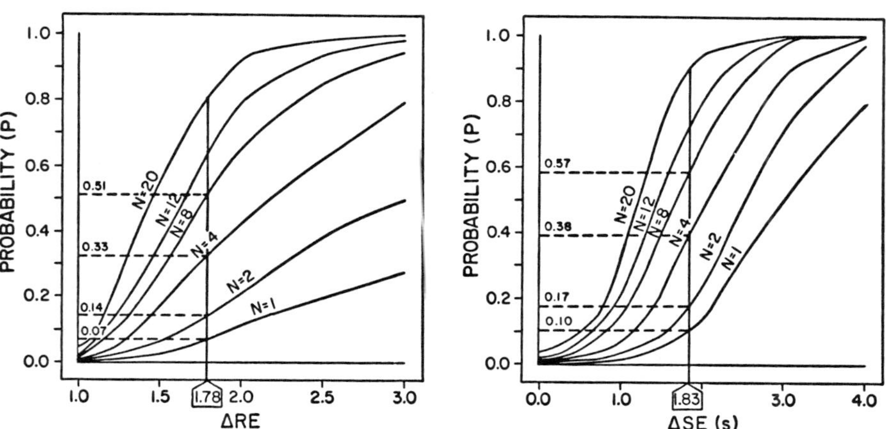

Fig. 3-5. Probability of rejection for analytical runs having medically important random error (*left,* ΔRE = 1.78) or systematic error (*right,* ΔSE = 1.83s) when using a Levey–Jennings control chart having ±3s control limits

ments would be required to have a 90% chance of detecting the critical systematic error.

From the power-function graphs for the Levey–Jennings control chart having ±2s control limits, the probability for false rejection is about 5% for N = 1, 10% for N = 2, and 18% for N = 4 (ARL_as of 1/0.05 = 20, 1/0.10 = 10, and 1/0.18 = 5.6, respectively). False rejections of 10 to 18% would seriously affect the productivity of the analytical process, wasting 10 to 18% of the production on repeat work. To determine the probabilities for detecting the critical random error, we draw a vertical line from 1.78 on the *x*-axis of the power-function graph for random error, as shown in Figure 3-6 (left). If the critical random error occurs, there is a 26% chance of detection when N = 1; 43% for N = 2; 75% for N = 4 (ARL_rs of 1/0.26 = 3.8, 1/0.43 = 2.3, and 1/0.75 = 1.3, respectively). To determine the probabilities for detecting the critical systematic error, we draw a vertical line from 1.83 on the *x*-axis of the power-function graph for systematic error, as shown in Figure 3-6 (right). If the critical systematic error occurs, there is a 42% chance of detection when N = 1; 67% when N = 2; 90% when N = 4 (ARL_rs of 1/0.42 = 2.4, 1/0.67 = 1.5, and 1/0.90 = 1.1, respectively).

In evaluating the performance of the Levey–Jennings control chart, the problem with the use of ±3s control limits is that the probability for error detection is very low, whereas the problem with the use of ±2s control limits is that the probability for false rejection is too high whenever N > 1.

In comparing the performance of the two control procedures, the

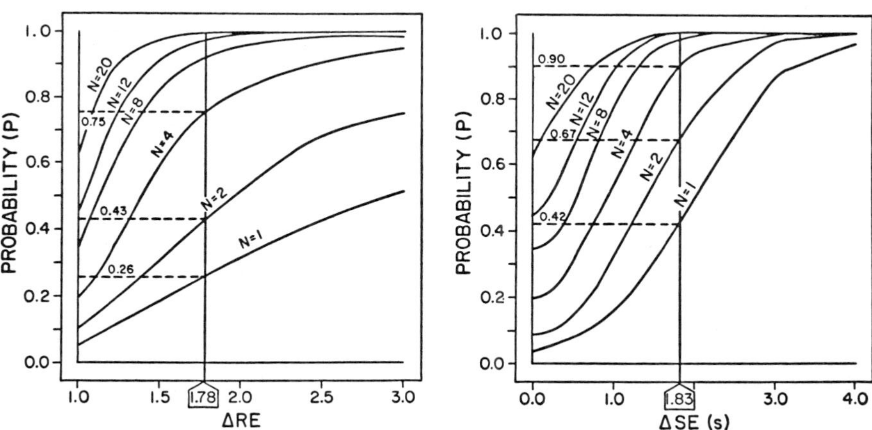

Fig. 3-6. Probability of rejection for analytical runs having medically important random error (*left,* ΔRE = 1.78) or systematic error (*right,* ΔSE = 1.83s) when using a Levey–Jennings control chart having ± 2s control limits

use of ±2s control limits with N = 1 gives about the same error detection (P_{ed} = 0.26 for ΔRE of 1.78, 0.42 for ΔSE of 1.83s) as the use of ±3s control limits with N = 4 (P_{ed} = 0.33 for ΔRE of 1.78, 0.38 for ΔSE of 1.83s). Although the quality of the two analytical processes would be nearly equivalent, the productivities of the two processes may differ: there would be a 5% false-rejection rate with the 1_{2s} control procedure, but only a 1% false-rejection rate with the 1_{3s} control procedure. The apparent 4% gain from the use of ±3s control limits would be offset by the need for four control measurements. To accurately predict the effect on the productivity of an analytical process, we must consider in more detail the type of measurement procedure and the relative numbers of patients' samples, calibrators, and control samples in each run. We will discuss these factors in more detail in Chapters 5 and 6.

Comparison of the Performance of Control Procedures

By comparing the power-function graphs for Levey–Jennings charts having ±2s and ±3s control limits, we have learned that there may be large differences in the probabilities for false rejection and error detection for different control procedures. Selection of control procedures should therefore be based on a careful comparison of the performance of the different control rules that may be used.

Power-function graphs and calculations of average run length provide the quantitative information for comparing the performance of control procedures. The power-function graphs by themselves are sufficient for assessing detection of intermittent errors, as well as persistent errors when a control procedure's probability for rejection does not change from run to run (which is true for Levey–Jennings charts having either ±2s or ±3s control limits). ARLs need to be calculated primarily when there are persistent errors and control procedures for which P_{ed} changes from run to run (see Chapter 4). For now, we will compare the performance of different control procedures by comparing probabilities for rejection.

In comparing control procedures, the one with the greatest P_{ed} and the lowest P_{fr} would generally be the best (putting aside for the moment any considerations of practicality and cost). Unfortunately, the choice is often more complicated than this because, for some control procedures, P_{ed} and P_{fr} are both higher. In such cases, the comparison should consider the acceptability of the false-rejection rate first and then the error-detection rate.

The need to keep the incidence of false rejections to an acceptable or tolerable rate can be explained by a simple analogy. A control system is an alarm system. Consider a fire-alarm system and what would happen if the fire alarm when off right now while you are reading this sentence. Most likely you would respond by moving to a safe location, away from the area of the fire. Suppose that, as you wait and wonder, someone arrives and informs you that there is no fire, that the alarm system has malfunctioned, that this was just a "false alarm." If you return to your task of reading, only to be interrupted again by an alarm, what would you do now? Would you again leave and move to a safe location? What if this happened a third time? How many false alarms would it take before you started to disregard the alarm system, attributing the problem to the alarm itself and no longer considering whether there really might be a cause for the alarm?

Because frequent false alarms will condition us to have a lack of response to all alarms, it is important in most situations to keep the incidence of false alarms low. Control procedures that do not meet this requirement for an acceptably low probability for false rejection are not generally useful in the laboratory. When P_{fr} is considered acceptably low (<0.05, or 5%), then the error detection of different control procedures or control rules can be compared.

Control Rules

Many different criteria can be used to interpret control data (*1*). As mentioned in Chapter 2, we use the term *control rule* to represent a decision criterion by which one interprets control data and makes a judgment on the control status of an analytical run. We symbolize these rules in the general form A_L, where A is the abbreviation for a particular statistic or is the number of control measurements, and L is the control limit. An analytical run is rejected when the control measurements fulfill the stated conditions, i.e., when a certain statistic or number of control measurements exceed specified limits. For example, 1_{2s} would be a control rule whereby a rejection is indicated when one control measurement (A = 1) exceeds $\bar{x} \pm 2s$ (L = 2s). 1_{2s} represents a Levey–Jennings chart having control limits set at $\bar{x} \pm 2s$, whereas 1_{3s} represents the Levey–Jennings chart having control limits at $\bar{x} \pm 3s$.

Among the control rules that have been used to interpret control data are the following:

1_{2s} One control measurement exceeds $\bar{x} \pm 2s$ (*6,7*). Historically, this was a "warning" limit on a Shewhart chart (*7*), but it is more often used in clinical laboratories as a rejection limit on a Levey–Jennings chart.

1_{3s} One control measurement exceeds $\bar{x} \pm 3s$ (*6,7*). This is the "action" or rejection limit recommended for a Shewhart control chart, and is similarly used on Levey–Jennings charts in clinical laboratories.

2_{2s} Two consecutive control measurements exceed the same limit, which is either $\bar{x} + 2s$ or $\bar{x} - 2s$ (*6*).

R_{4s} The difference between the high and low control measurements within a run exceeds 4s (*8*).

3_{1s} Three consecutive control measurements exceed the same limit, which is either $\bar{x} + 1s$ or $\bar{x} - 1s$ (*9*).

4_{1s} Four consecutive control measurements exceed the same limit, which is either $\bar{x} + 1s$ or $\bar{x} - 1s$ (*6*).

$7_{\bar{x}}$ Seven consecutive control measurements fall on one side of the mean (*6,10*).

7_T Seven consecutive control measurements show a trend upwards, or downwards (*10*).

$10_{\bar{x}}$ Ten consecutive control measurements fall on one side of the mean (*9*).

$1_{P_{fr}}$ One control measurement in a group of N control measurements exceeds control limits that have been chosen to have a specified probability for false rejection, P_{fr}. For example, $1_{0.05}$ would be a control rule having limits chosen to maintain a 0.05 probability for false rejection. The control limits change with N, widening as N increases (see Table AI-2 in Appendix I for factors for calculating the control limits).

$2_{P_{fr}}$ Two consecutive control measurements in a group of N control measurements exceed the same control limit, which is chosen to have a specified probability for false rejection, P_{fr}. For example, $2_{0.05}$ is a control rule having limits chosen to maintain a 0.05 probability for false rejection. The control limits change with N, widening as N increases (see Table AI-2, Appendix I).

The above control rules apply to "individual-value control charts," for which individual control measurements can be plotted and interpreted directly. When the control measurements are subjected to prior calculations, with the resulting control statistics being plotted and interpreted, other control charts are used, such as cumulative sum, mean, range, and standard deviation charts. The following symbols are used to represent control rules for these kinds of charts:

CS The differences between the individual control measurements and $\bar{x}$ are calculated and summed to give the total or cumulative sum. The "cusum" is then judged by graphical techniques, e.g., **V**-mask cusum (*11*), or by numerical control limits, e.g., decision limit cusum (*12*).

$\bar{x}_{P_{fr}}$ The mean of a group of N control measurements exceeds control limits having a specified probability for false rejection, P_{fr} (*7,13*). For example, $\bar{x}_{0.05}$ would be a "mean rule" with control limits chosen to maintain a 0.05 probability of false rejection. The actual limits decrease as N increases, so as to keep P_{fr} constant (see Table AI-2 in Appendix I).

$R_{P_{fr}}$ The range, or difference between the high and low measurements in a group of N control measurements, exceeds an upper one-sided control limit having a specified probability for false rejection, P_{fr} (*7,13*). For example, $R_{0.05}$ would be a "range rule" with control limits chosen to maintain a 0.05 probability of false rejection. The actual control limits increase as N increases, so as to keep P_{fr} constant (see Table AI-2).

$\chi^2_{P_{fr}}$ The ratio s^2_{obs} $(N - 1)/s^2$ exceeds the critical chi-square value having a specified P_{fr}, where s_{obs} is the standard deviation observed (or calculated) from the control measurements and s is the stable standard deviation of the measurement procedure (*14*). For example, $\chi^2_{0.05}$ is a "chi-square rule" with control limits chosen to maintain a 0.05 probability of false rejection. The critical chi-square value varies with N and with the chosen P_{fr} (see Table AI-2).

Response Curves

To illustrate the false-rejection and error-detection characteristics of commonly used control rules, let us consider the responses of different control rules as a function of the number of control observations per run (N). We call these plots or lines "response curves" to distinguish them from "power curves." Response curves show the probability for rejection for a specified error condition as a function of the number of control measurements, whereas power curves show the probability for rejection for a specified number of control measurements as a function of the size of the analytical error. Response curves are useful for comparing the performance of different control procedures for a given error condition. One can construct reponse curves from power-function graphs by selecting a single error condition (i.e., picking a value on the *x*-axis), then plotting the probability for rejection vs N. For example, a response curve illustrating the false rejections for the 1_{2s} control rule can be obtained from the information in Figure 3-2 or 3-3 by plotting the *y*-intercept values (P_{fr}) vs the respective N values for each power curve. In constructing response curves, one may choose to have the *y*-axis represent values for *P*, P_{fr}, or P_{ed}, depending on what error conditions are being compared.

Figure 3-7 allows comparison of the false-rejection probabilities of different control rules for a wide range of N. The error condition of interest is "no errors" except for the inherent imprecision of the measurement procedure. Clearly, as N increases, the false rejections increase, particularly for the 1_{2s}, 3_{1s}, and $7_{\bar{x}}$ control rules. For low values of N, false rejection is perhaps not much of a problem for the 3_{1s}

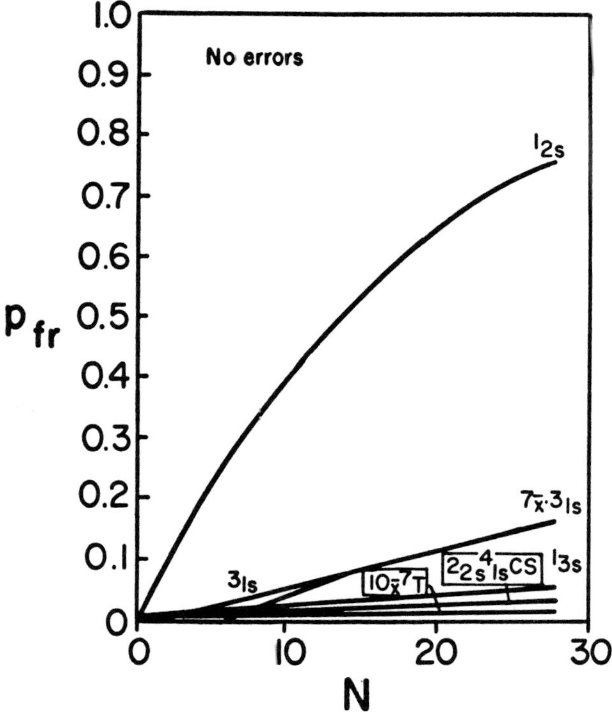

Fig. 3-7. Responses of control rules when there are no analytical errors present except for the inherent imprecision of the measurement procedure

From Westgard et al. (*1*), reprinted with permission

and $7_{\bar{x}}$ rules, but if those rules are applied to the review of monthly control charts having 20 to 30 plotted points, then the false rejections are of greater concern. All the other commonly used control rules (that are included in the discussion here) provide acceptably low rates of false rejection.

To compare the error-detection probabilities of various control rules, we will simplify the interpretation by confining our evaluation to the response curves for rules having acceptably low (<5%) false-rejection rates. This limitation applies mainly to the 1_{2s} control rule. For example, Figure 3-8 shows the probability for rejection of the 1_{2s} control rule for a ΔRE of 1.5 (50% increase in the standard deviation of the measurement procedure). The apparent error-detection rate (the upper curve) may be misleading if the false-rejection rate (the lower curve) is not considered. The true error detection is the difference between the

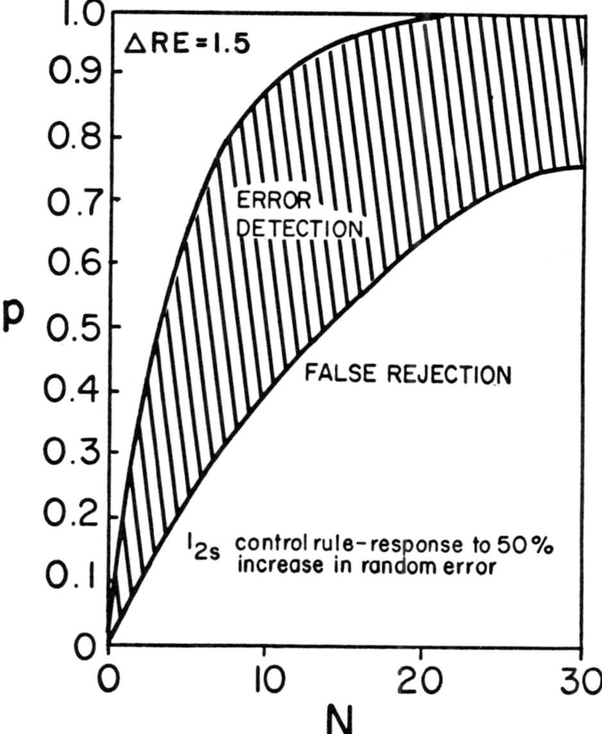

Fig. 3-8. The probabilities of false rejection and error detection for a Levey–Jennings control chart having ±2s control limits (1_{2s} control rule) as a function of the number of control measurements (N)

The *shaded area* corresponds to the true probability for detection of errors

two lines. Because of this complication, we have not included the 1_{2s} rule in the following figures.

The upper panels of Figure 3-9 show the probability for detecting a 50% increase in random error (ΔRE = 1.5) for the control rules having low false-rejection rates. Note the differences in the sensitivities of the different control rules. Of the simpler control rules, the 1_{3s} rule is more sensitive than the 2_{2s} rule, which, in turn, is more sensitive than the 4_{1s} and the $10_{\bar{x}}$ rules. In general, the error detection of range (R-chart) and chi-square (S-chart) rules is greater than that of the other rules. Note also that as the probability for false rejection is allowed to increase from 0.002 to 0.01 to 0.05, the error detection improves, as would be expected.

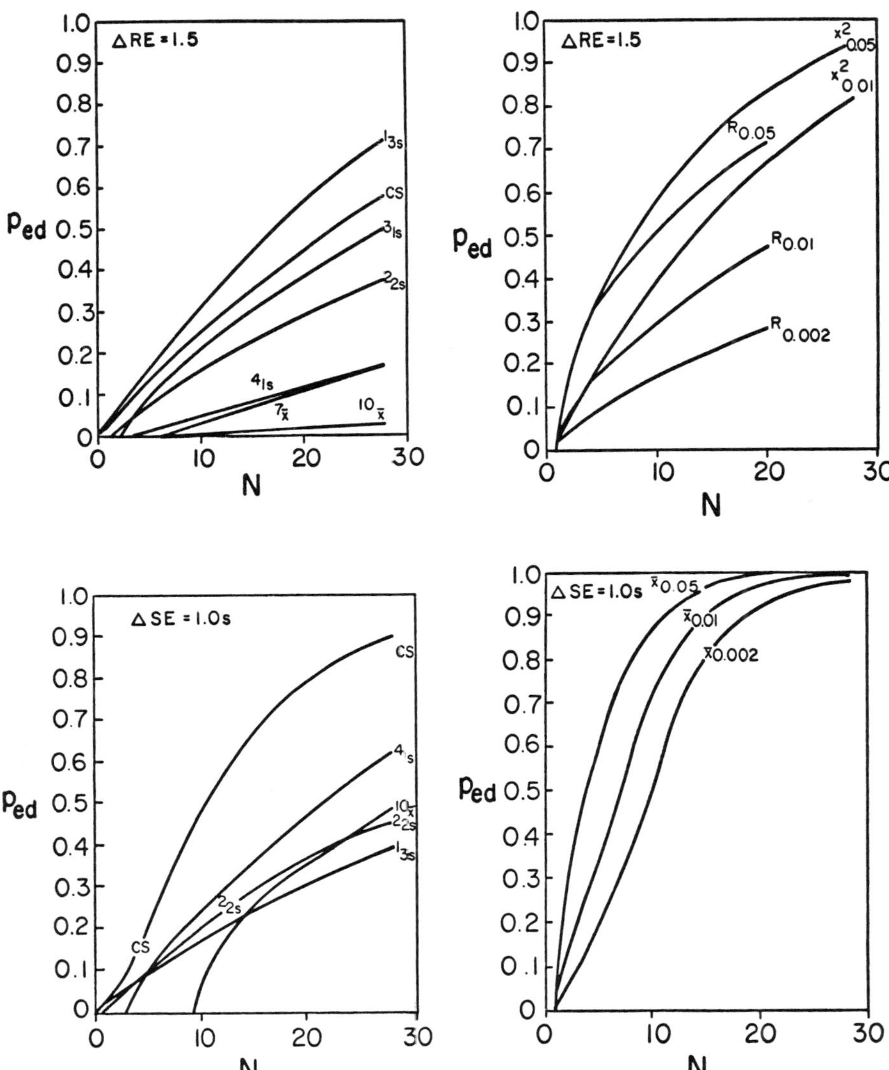

Fig. 3-9. *Upper panels,* responses of control rules to an increase in random error (ΔRE = 1.5); *lower panels,* responses of control rules to a systematic error (ΔSE = 1.0s)

From Westgard et al. (*1*), reprinted with permission

The responses to systematic errors ($\Delta SE = 1.0s$) are shown in the lower panels of Figure 3-9. Observe that the 4_{1s}, 2_{2s}, and $10_{\bar{x}}$ rules are more sensitive to systematic errors than is the 1_{3s} rule. Rules requiring consecutive measurements on one side of a control limit are more responsive to systematic error than to random error. Cusum rules have a high rate of error detection because of the cumulative use of all of the control measurements. Rules based on the mean of a group of control measurements are likewise more sensitive than rules for individual value charts, probably because they make more quantitative use of all of the control measurements.

From such comparisons, we can make the following general assessment of the performance characteristics of control rules. When there are no errors present, the 1_{2s}, 3_{1s}, and $7_{\bar{x}}$ rules tend to have too high P_{fr}. When there are random errors present, the rules with the highest P_{ed} are the 1_{3s} rule for individual value charts, the $R_{0.05}$ and $R_{0.01}$ rules for range charts, and the $\chi^2_{0.05}$ and $\chi^2_{0.01}$ rules for S-charts. When there are systematic errors present, the rules with the highest P_{ed} are the 2_{2s}, 4_{1s}, and $10_{\bar{x}}$ rules for individual value charts, the $\bar{x}_{0.05}$ and $\bar{x}_{0.01}$ rules for mean charts, and the CS rule for a cusum chart.

Implications for the Selection or Design of Control Procedures

With an understanding of the performance characteristics of statistical control procedures and with some knowledge of the performance of different control rules, we can now start to consider what should be done to select or design cost-effective quality-control procedures.

Select or design on the basis of performance characteristics. Control rules should be chosen to have a low probability for false rejection (P_{fr}) and a high probability for error detection (P_{ed}). Because the 1_{2s}, 3_{1s}, and $7_{\bar{x}}$ rules may generate a high rate of false rejections, their use must be carefully considered. It would generally be safest to avoid them unless a specific application requires a very high rate of error detection and the expense of false rejections is not a limitation. For detection of random error, the 1_{3s}, range, and chi-square rules provide the best sensitivity. For detection of systematic error, the 2_{2s}, 4_{1s}, $10_{\bar{x}}$, mean, and cusum rules provide best error detection.

In general, P_{ed} will increase as P_{fr} increases; i.e., a control procedure will detect more errors when the rate of false rejections is allowed to increase. P_{ed} will also increase as the number of control observations (N) increases, and so might P_{fr} unless the control limits are adjusted to take N into account (e.g., the $1_{0.05}$, $2_{0.05}$ types of rules).

Define a tolerable false-rejection rate. One of the first decisions to make when selecting or designing a control procedure is what value of P_{fr} is tolerable or acceptable. In industrial applications, probabilities as low as 0.002 are often selected because the cost of rejecting a run is very high, in terms of both the materials lost and the time required to investigate the process, correct the disturbance, and re-start the process. These costs are also appreciable in clinical laboratories, but the runs often take only a short time and the process often is very rapid and easily re-started. Consequently, it should be possible to tolerate higher P_{fr} values, and thereby gain improved error detection.

Values for P_{fr} in the range of 0.01 to 0.05 seem reasonable in view of the effort already routinely expended for quality control in clinical laboratories. A value of 0.05 implies a 5.0% loss in productivity for the analytical process, caused by repeating the analyses for those samples in analytical runs that are judged to be out-of-control, but does not consider other losses for investigating the process and correcting any disturbances. Such a loss in the productivity of an analytical process may be tolerable in laboratories having excess capacity, but others may prefer to choose a more conservative value (e.g., 0.01) for the false-rejection rate. The efforts expended in routine repetition would be better applied to improving the performance of the control procedure—most easily by increasing N, but also by adopting more sensitive control rules. The goal is to achieve the highest error detection with the least loss in the productivity of the analytical process.

There may, of course, be situations where it is difficult to achieve the rate of error detection and the quality desired without letting the rate of false rejections increase. If it is not practical to increase N or to change to more complicated control statistics, the use of simple control rules with high rates of false rejections may provide the necessary error detection. The costs of such procedures, however, should be fully understood, both for their impact on productivity (the portion of the workload that will be repeated) and for the possible impact of the many false alarms on the laboratory analysts.

Consider control rules having a specified false-rejection rate. The main limitation of a Levey–Jennings chart with ±2s control limits is its high probability for false rejection when N is 2 or greater. Figure 3-10 shows the probability for false rejection as a function of N, illustrating how high P_{fr} gets as N increases. A chart having ±3s control limits reduces the number of false rejections, but has a relatively low probability for error detection. Widening control limits from ±2s to ±3s reduces both the false-rejection rate and the error-detection rate. To compensate for the low error-detection rate, the number of control measurements can be increased, but obtaining a high error-detection rate when ±3s control limits are used will require making many control measurements.

There is no reason why control limits have to be chosen only as ±2s or ±3s, except for the convenience of using integral multiples

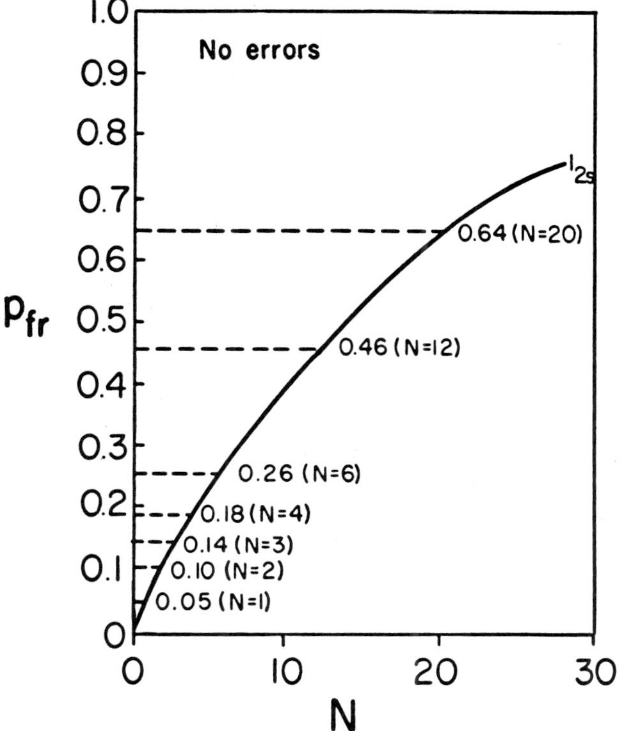

Fig. 3-10. Probability for false rejection for a Levey–Jennings control chart having ±2s control limits (1_{2s} control rule) as a function of the number of control measurements (N)

of s for manual calculations and manual implementation of the control procedures. Control limits could instead be chosen at other multiples of s if desirable, to fix the false rejections at a specified probability. One could have the control limits vary as N changes, to keep P_{fr} constant, rather than fix the control limits and have P_{fr} vary as N changes.

Use of control rules such as $1_{0.05}$, $1_{0.01}$, or $1_{0.002}$ may improve performance, keeping false rejections at a tolerable level and gaining maximum error detection. Table AI-2 (Appendix I) summarizes the factors for calculating control limits for these rules for different numbers of control measurements per run (N).

As an example of how to use the factors in Table AI-2, consider what control limits should be used to keep false rejections at 1% when there are two to four control measurements per run. From the row in the table for the $1_{0.01}$ control rule, and the columns where N = 2 and N = 4, we can see that the control limits would be set as $\bar{x} \pm$ 2.81s for N = 2; for N = 4, they would be $\bar{x} \pm$ 3.01s. Thus, the control procedure should have control limits of 2.81s when N = 2 and 3.01s when N = 4. Note that as N increases, the control limits widen to keep the false-rejection rate constant.

One use of this kind of control procedure would be to provide maximum error detection with a single control rule, while keeping false rejections at a chosen tolerable rate. Rather than switching from ±2s to ±3s control limits when N is 2 or greater, one could improve error detection by using a $1_{0.05}$ control rule (2.24s control limits at N = 2) or a $1_{0.01}$ control rule (2.81s control limits at N = 2). The narrower control limits would give better error detection, while maintaining a tolerable rate of false rejections.

Another use could be to minimize the false-rejection rate on simultaneous multi-channel analyzers. As the number of channels increases, use of fixed control limits causes an increase in the false rejections, just as if N were increasing. In fact, N is increasing, but it is the total N for the analyzer, not the N per channel. For example, for a six-channel analyzer having one control measurement per channel, use of 2s control limits would cause approximately one run out of four to have a false-rejection signal on at least one channel. To maintain a 5% false-rejection rate for the analyzer as a whole, control limits could be set as $\bar{x} \pm$ 2.64s on each channel. For a six-channel analyzer having two control measurements per channel per run, a 5% false-rejection rate would require control limits to be set ± 2.86s from the mean (for each channel). Note again that the control limits get wider as the numbers of channels and control measurements increase, resulting in a lower rate of error detection per channel.

The performance expected for rules of this type can be found in Appendix II. Such rules have not been applied to any great extent in clinical laboratories, probably because of the difficulties of explaining why the control charts have different control limits when N changes. With more widespread use of computers in quality control, more applications of such rules can be expected.

Assess error detection for medically important errors. In comparing the performance of different control procedures, we assess the error-detection capabilities for the medically important random and systematic errors. The size of the critical random and systematic errors can be calculated as described in Chapter 2 (equations 2-3 and 2-7). In the absence of such calculations, consider the following errors to be important: an increase in random error corresponding to a doubling of the stable standard deviation (s) (ΔRE = 2.0) and a systematic shift equivalent to two times the size of s (ΔSE = 2.0s).

Develop multi-rule control procedures to increase error detection. From the observed performance of the different control rules we have considered, we can take another approach to improving the performance of control procedures. Because no single control rule provides the best sensitivity to both random and systematic errors, it is desirable that a control procedure use some combination of rules—some rules sensitive to random error and some sensitive to systematic error. One approach for developing a suitable combination of rules is as follows:

1. From the control rules being considered, eliminate those having a high probability for false rejection.
2. From the remaining rules, select at least one that is sensitive to random error and one that is sensitive to systematic error.
3. Assess the performance of this combination by using power-function graphs and ARL calculations.
4. Select the number of control observations that will give an appropriate probability for detecting the errors of interest.

From the earlier categorization of control rules, several combinations of rules could be suggested. After eliminating the high-P_{fr} group of rules, select at least one rule from the high-P_{ed} groups for random and systematic errors. For simple control charts, a 1_{3s} rule could be used for random error and a 2_{2s} rule for systematic error. Other rules could be added to improve error detection, such as a range rule for random error, plus the 4_{1s} and (or) $10_{\bar{x}}$ rule for systematic error. When more complicated calculations can be implemented, charts based on mean and range (or chi-square) rules should be useful. Cusum charts could also be used, but should be coupled with an additional control rule for detecting random error. Some example multi-rule control procedures are discussed in detail in Chapter 4.

Summary

The performance of a control procedure can be assessed quantitatively by using terms for probability for rejection (P) or for average run length (ARL). When analytical errors are *intermittent,* the critical performance characteristics are the probability for false rejection (P_{fr}) and the probability for error detection (P_{ed}). These characteristics describe the portion of analytical runs that will be rejected when different amounts of analytical error are present. When analytical errors are *persistent,* the critical characteristics are the average run length for acceptable quality (ARL_a) and the average run length for rejectable quality (ARL_r). These characteristics describe how many runs will occur before a run is rejected.

Information on probabilities for rejection can be obtained from computer simulation studies and can be displayed in power-function graphs: plots of the probability for rejection vs the size of analytical error (either random error or systematic error). The probability for false rejection is given by the y-intercept. The probability for error detection can be assessed for different sizes of errors, as appropriate for the specific analytical process under consideration. Average run lengths can be calculated from these probabilities.

Different control procedures or control rules have different probabilities for false rejection, as well as different probabilities for error detection. Because of this, the quality and productivity of an analytical process will be affected by the control rules chosen. Control procedures should be selected on the basis of a low P_{fr} and a high P_{ed}.

In selecting or designing a control procedure, analysts should first consider the probability for false rejection, keeping it low to minimize problems in reacting to "false alarms." Control rules having a high probability of false rejections should generally be eliminated, unless there are special circumstances that require a high rate of error detection at the expense of many false rejections. Achieving the high error detection may require increasing the number of control measurements, using a control rule with a specified P_{fr}, or using control procedures with more than one decision criterion (multi-rule procedures).

The selection and design of control procedures should be based on careful consideration of their performance characteristics. Appendix II presents power-function graphs for many of the control rules commonly used in clinical laboratories. For new or modified control procedures, computer simulation programs provide a practical way of making this information available to laboratory managers and analysts.

References

1. Westgard JO, Groth T, Aronsson T, Falk H, de Verdier C-H. Performance characteristics of rules for internal quality control: probabilities for false rejection and error detection. Clin Chem 1977;23:1857–67.

2. Groth T, Falk H, Westgard JO. An interactive computer simulation program for the design of statistical control procedures in clinical chemistry. Comput Programs Biomed 1981;13:73–86.

3. Westgard JO, Groth T. Design and evaluation of statistical control procedures: applications of a computer "Quality Control Simulator" program. Clin Chem 1981;27:1536–45.

4. Westgard JO, Falk H, Groth T. Influence of a between-run component of variation, choice of control limits, and shape of error distribution on the performance characteristics of rules for internal quality control. Clin Chem 1979;25:394–400.

5. Westgard JO, Groth T. Power functions for statistical control rules. Clin Chem 1979;25:863–9.

6. Duncan AJ. Quality control and industrial statistics, 4th ed. Homewood, IL: Richard D Irwin, Inc., 1974:392.

7. Shewhart WA. Economic control of quality of the manufactured product. New York: Van Nostrand, 1931.

8. Westgard JO, Barry PL, Hunt MR, Groth T. A multi-rule Shewhart chart for quality control in clinical chemistry. Clin Chem 1981;27:493–501.

9. Jardine AKS, MacFarlane JD, Greensted CS. Statistical methods for quality control. Bath, U.K.: The Pitman Press, 1975:133.

10. Stamm D. Introduction of quality control for all quantitative clinical chemical analyses in West Germany. Dtsch Ges Klin Chem Mitt 1974;2:25.

11. Davies OL, Goldsmith PL. Statistical methods in research and production, 4th ed. New York: Hafner Publishing Co., 1972:401–8.

12. Westgard JO, Groth T, Aronsson T, de Verdier C-H. A combined Shewhart-cusum control chart for improved quality control in clinical chemistry. Clin Chem 1977;23:1881–7.

13. Op. cit. (ref. *6*):431–51.

14. Ostle BA. Statistics in research, 2nd ed. Ames, IA: The Iowa State College Press, 1954:87.

CHAPTER 4

Improving Quality Control by the Use of Multi-Rule Control Procedures

In clinical laboratories, individual control measurements are usually plotted directly on control charts, e.g., the Levey–Jennings chart in Chapter 2. The control limits are usually set as the mean ± 2s or the mean ± 3s (1_{2s} or 1_{3s} control rules) to determine whether an analytical run should be accepted (an in-control run) or rejected (an out-of-control run).

In Chapter 3, we described the performance of Levey–Jennings control charts and observed that Levey–Jennings charts with ±2s control limits lead to too many false rejections when there are two or more control measurements per run. False rejections reduce the productivity of an analytical process because analytical results are discarded and new runs performed to analyze those same patients' samples again, even though there are no errors except for the inherent imprecision of the measurement procedure. Levey–Jennings charts with ±3s control limits reduce the false rejections, but also reduce the error detection, potentially affecting the quality of an analytical process by allowing defects (analytical errors) to go undetected. Error detection can be increased by increasing the number of control measurements per run (N), which consumes more of the process output for analyzing control samples and reduces productivity.

Another approach for improving error detection is to select "multi-rule" rather than "single-rule" control procedures. In multi-rule control procedures, two or more control rules are used for testing control measurements and determining control status. Each control rule is chosen because it has a low probability for false rejection and as high a probability for error detection as possible. A well-chosen combination of control rules can increase the probability for error detection, thus improving error detection without requiring a higher number of control measurements. Well-designed multi-rule control procedures will be cost-effective if they can provide improved quality without the increased costs (and lower productivity) from additional control measurements.

A widely used multi-rule control procedure is the one recommended by Westgard et al. as a Selected Method in clinical chemistry (*1*). In this chapter we will describe that multi-rule procedure, present its performance characteristics, and compare its performance with other individual-value control procedures. However, it is important to understand that "multi-rule" quality control is a concept, not a specific control procedure. There are other applications in clinical laboratories (*2–5*) and similar applications in industry (*6,7*), although industry is more likely to apply the rules to the means of groups of control measurements rather than to individual control measurements.

Westgard Multi-Rule Control Procedure

The objectives in developing this control procedure were to provide: (*a*) simple data analysis and display via individual-value control charts; (*b*) easy adaptation and integration into existing control practices based on Levey–Jennings charts; (*c*) a low probability for false rejections or false alarms; (*d*) an improved capability for detecting analytical errors; and (*e*) some indication of the type of analytical error occurring when a run is rejected, to aid in problem-solving and resolution of out-of-control situations (*1*).

Westgard Rules

Six control rules are recommended (*1*). Commonly known as "Westgard rules," they are defined as follows:

1_{2s} represents the control rule whereby one control measurement exceeding control limits of $\bar{x} \pm 2s$ provides a "warning." It is interpreted as a requirement for additional inspection of the control data by testing with the other rules to judge whether the analytical run should be accepted or rejected.

1_{3s} is the control rule whereby a run is rejected when one control measurement exceeds control limits set at $\bar{x} \pm 3s$. This rule is primarily sensitive to random error, but also responds to large systematic errors.

2_{2s} is the control rule whereby the run is rejected when two consecutive control measurements exceed the same limit, which is either $\bar{x} + 2s$ or $\bar{x} - 2s$. The rule is initially applied to measurements within a run. Both measurements can be on the same control material ("within material"), or there can be one measurement on two different control materials ("across materials"). A run is rejected when two consecutive control measurements within the run exceed their respective +2s control limits or their respective −2s control limits. When applied to consecutive measurements on different materials ("across materials"), the rule is sensitive to systematic errors occurring throughout the analytical range being tested. When applied to consecutive measurements on the same material ("within material"), the rule is sensitive to systematic errors occurring at one concentration. The rule can also be applied to two consecutive measurements on the same material, one from each of two consecutive runs ("within material, across runs").

R_{4s} is the control rule whereby a run is rejected when the range or difference between the high and low control measurements within a run exceeds 4s. For manual implementations, the rule can be invoked when one measurement within the run exceeds the +2s limit and the other exceeds the −2s limit. For computer implementations, the rule can be invoked in a more quantitative manner, taking the exact difference between the high and low measurements in the run. This rule is sensitive to random errors.

4_{1s} is the control rule whereby a run is rejected when four consecutive control measurements exceed the same limit, either $\bar{x} + 1s$ or $\bar{x} - 1s$. The consecutive measurements can occur within one control material, which may require inspecting the measurements for a single material from up to four consecutive runs, or the measurements can occur "across" control materials, reducing the number of runs required to accumulate four measurements. This rule is sensitive to systematic errors.

$10_{\bar{x}}$ is the control rule that requires 10 consecutive control measurements to fall on one side of the mean. The measurements will occur over several runs, and can be assessed within or across control materials. The rule is sensitive to systematic errors.

A practical way of using this combination of control rules in a manual application is shown in Figure 4-1. The 1_{2s} rule is used as a warning rule to trigger a detailed inspection of the control data with the other control rules. If no control measurement exceeds a 2s limit, the analytical run is judged in-control and the patients' data may be reported. If a control measurement exceeds a 2s limit, the control data are tested further by applying the 1_{3s}, 2_{2s}, R_{4s}, 4_{1s}, and $10_{\bar{x}}$ rules. If none of these rules are violated, the run is in control. If any one rule is violated, then the run is out of control. The particular rule violated may give some indication of the type of analytical error occurring. Random error will often be detected by the 1_{3s} or R_{4s} rules, whereas systematic error will usually be detected by the 2_{2s}, 4_{1s}, or $10_{\bar{x}}$ rules and, when very large, by the 1_{3s} rule.

Preparation of Control Charts

Control limits can be calculated from monthly data or from cumulative data, as illustrated earlier in Chapter 2. Limits are needed for $\bar{x} \pm 1s$, $\bar{x} \pm 2s$, and $\bar{x} \pm 3s$. Of the many different kinds of charts or records one can prepare for manual use of the multi-rule procedure, three possibilities are illustrated here. The choice between them depends on how many control materials are used, the relative frequency

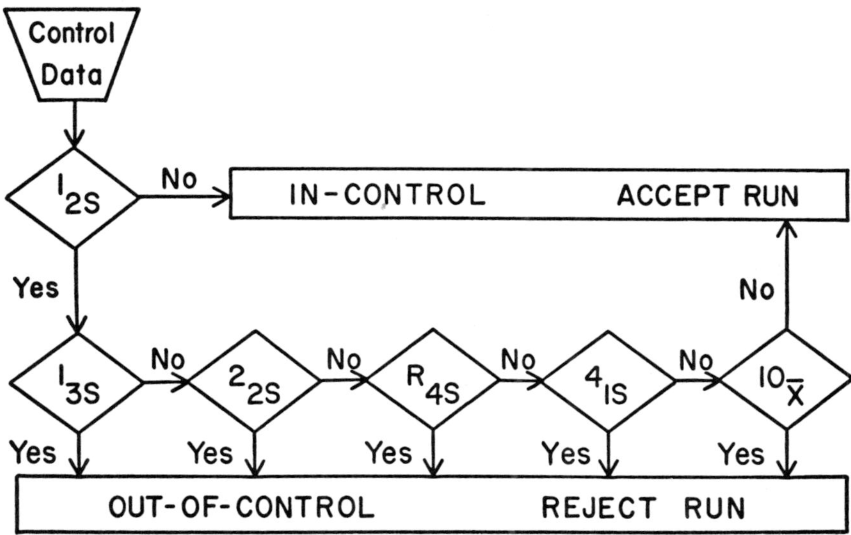

Fig. 4-1. Logic diagram for applying the $1_{3s}/2_{2s}/R_{4s}/4_{1s}/10_{\bar{x}}$ series of control rules in a multi-rule control procedure

From Westgard et al. (*1*), reprinted with permission

of use of each control material, and whether there is a preference for control charts or tabular records.

Control charts for individual materials. For each control material, prepare a control chart by scaling the *y*-axis to provide a concentration range from $\bar{x} - 4s$ to $\bar{x} + 4s$ and scaling the *x*-axis to provide the time period of interest. Label the *y*-axis in terms of concentration units and the *x*-axis by either date or run number. Horizontal lines should be drawn corresponding to $\bar{x}$, $\bar{x} \pm 1s$, $\bar{x} \pm 2s$, and $\bar{x} \pm 3s$ (see Figure 4-2 for an example). The control limits can be color-coded for easier use; e.g., green for $\bar{x}$, blue for $\bar{x} \pm 1s$, orange for $\bar{x} \pm 2s$, and red for $\bar{x} \pm 3s$.

Tabular charts. For some manual applications, a tabular record may be as convenient as a control chart. One could use a recording form with the following columns: $<\bar{x} - 3s$; $\bar{x} - 3s$ to $\bar{x} - 2s$; $\bar{x} - 2s$ to $\bar{x} - 1s$; $\bar{x} - 1s$ to $\bar{x}$; $\bar{x}$ to $\bar{x} + 1s$; $\bar{x} + 1s$ to $\bar{x} + 2s$; $\bar{x} + 2s$ to $\bar{x} + 3s$; $>\bar{x} + 3s$. Lines could be drawn between the columns to represent limit lines and could be color-coded like the limit lines on a multi-rule chart (see Figure 4-3).

The numerical values of the control measurements, when entered in the appropriate columns, provide both a record and a display of the control results. The primary difference from a control chart is that the time axis runs vertically; in effect, the control chart is rotated

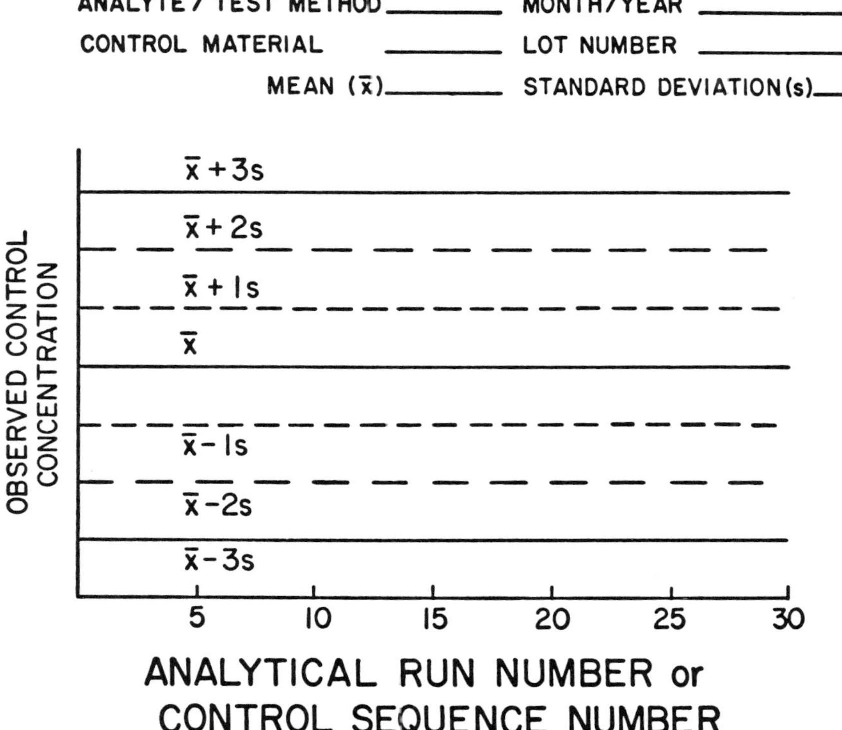

Fig. 4-2. Multi-rule control chart for use with individual control materials
From Westgard et al. (*1*), reprinted with permission

a quarter turn so that time runs down the page rather than across the page. By using this kind of tabular chart, one can record the accept or reject decision for each analytical run, along with documentation of any problems and their resolution.

z-score charts. To make it easier to keep track of the order of measurements when control materials are analyzed with different frequencies, prepare a single chart to display the "z-scores" for all the control measurements. A "z-score" is the difference between the control measurement and its respective mean, divided by the standard deviation for that control material:

$$z\text{-score} = (x_{i_{mat}} - \bar{x}_{mat})/s_{mat}$$

where the subscript refers to a particular control material, $x_{i_{mat}}$ is the ith measurement on a given material, $\bar{x}_{mat}$ is the mean for that material,

ANALYTE/TEST METHOD ________ MONTH/YEAR ________

CONTROL MATERIAL ________ LOT NUMBER ________

MEAN ($\bar{x}$) ________ STANDARD DEVIATION (s) ____

Run# Seq#	<-3s	-3s	-2s	-1s	$\bar{x}$	+1s	+2s	+3s	>+3s	Accept or Reject	Comments

Fig. 4-3. Tabular control chart and record

and s_{mat} is the stable standard deviation for that material. For example, if the control value of 124 is determined for a control material having a mean value of 120 and a standard deviation of 4, the *z*-score would be +1. A control chart for *z*-scores should be scaled from −4 to +4, with the mean being 0 and the limit lines being ±1, ±2, and ±3. The results for different control materials can be charted by using symbols or letters to represent each material. See Figure 4-4 for an example.

Any value on the *z*-score chart corresponds to the number of standard deviations that a measurement is from the mean of its respective control material. For example, a value of +1 would indicate that a control measurement was one standard deviation from the mean on that particular control material. Any four values in a row exceeding the +1 line would indicate a violation of the 4_{1s} rule, regardless of the order of the materials or their relative frequency of use.

Step-by-Step Multi-Rule Control Procedure for N = 2

The following details of the operation of a multi-rule control procedure describe an application having two control measurements (N = 2). The two measurements can be obtained from measurements made within a day, a shift, or a run, whatever is appropriate for the measure-

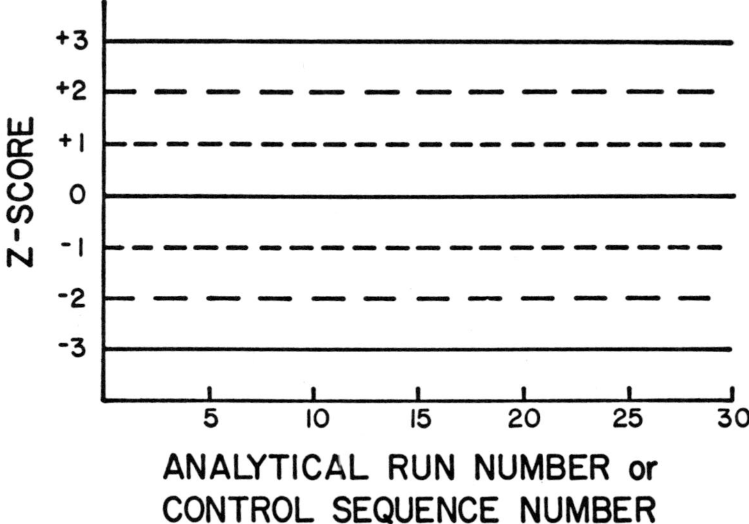

Fig. 4-4. *Z*-score control chart for use with two or more control materials

ment procedure being monitored. Recommendations on the locations, sequences, intervals, or times depend on the particular measurement procedure and the laboratory application. It may sometimes be appropriate to assign the control samples to random positions in a run; at other times, it may be desirable to place them in specific locations that bracket patients' samples. In some situations control samples may be analyzed before patients' samples, to establish that a measurement procedure is in a state of statistical control before proceeding with the analysis.

1. Analyze samples of two different control materials. Make one measurement on each control material each time when testing for statistical control. Record these measurements and plot them on the respective control charts for the two control materials.

2. Test the control data by using the 1_{2s} control rule. Accept the run when both control measurements are within $\bar{x} \pm 2s$ limits; report the patients' results. When at least one control measurement exceeds the $\bar{x} \pm 2s$ limits, withhold reporting of patients' results and inspect the control data further, using the additional control rules.

3. Inspect control data within the run.

a. Test with the 1_{3s} rule. Reject the run when one control measurement exceeds $\bar{x} \pm 3s$ limits; do not report patients' results.

b. Test with the 2_{2s} rule across control materials. Reject the run when both control measurements exceed the same $\bar{x} + 2s$ or $\bar{x} - 2s$ control limit; do not report patients' results.

c. Test with the R_{4s} rule, within the run, across control materials. Reject the run when one control measurement exceeds a $\bar{x} + 2s$ limit and the other exceeds a $\bar{x} - 2s$ limit; do not report patients' results.

4. Inspect control data across runs.

a. Test with the 2_{2s} rule within the control materials. Reject when the previous measurement on the same control material exceeds the same $\bar{x} + 2s$ or $\bar{x} - 2s$ control limit; do not report patients' results.

b. Test with the 4_{1s} rule across control materials. Reject when the last four consecutive control measurements exceed the same $\bar{x} + 1s$ or $\bar{x} - 1s$ limit; do not report patients' results.

c. Test with the 4_{1s} rule within control materials. Reject when the last four control measurements on the same control material exceed the same $\bar{x} + 1s$ or $\bar{x} - 1s$ control limit; do not report patients' results.

d. Test with the $10_{\bar{x}}$ rule across control materials. Reject when the last 10 consecutive control measurements fall on the same side of $\bar{x}$; do not report patients' results.

e. Test with the $10_{\bar{x}}$ rule within control materials. Reject when the last 10 measurements on the same control material fall on the same side of $\bar{x}$; do not report patients' results.

5. Accept the run when none of the rules indicates a lack of statistical control. Report patients' results.

6. When the analytical process is out of control:

a. Determine the type of errors occurring (random or systematic), on the basis of the control rules that are violated. When either the 1_{3s} or R_{4s} control rule is violated, the error is more likely random than systematic. When systematic error is present, it is more likely to be detected by the 2_{2s}, 4_{1s}, or $10_{\bar{x}}$ rules. A review of control data on both control materials (across materials) will help detect errors occurring throughout the concentration range tested by those control materials. A review of control data on a single control material (within material) will help detect errors occurring in a particular concentration range.

b. Refer to a troubleshooting guide to inspect the components of the measurement procedure that contribute to the type of error observed.

c. Correct the problem, then re-analyze the control and patients' samples, testing for statistical control by the same procedure. In assessing the control of the new run, do not include the control data from a previously rejected run.

d. Consult a supervisor for any decision to report data when there is a lack of statistical control (i.e., when any of the control rules gives a rejection signal).

7. One may decide to report patients' results when there is a lack of statistical control, in the following situations:

a. The control problem can be shown to be due to the control materials themselves.

b. The control problem can be shown to have resulted from an isolated event that would not have affected the rest of the run (e.g., an interchange of two control samples or a clerical transcription error).

c. The control problem occurs in a concentration range that is different from the concentrations of the patients' samples, and the analytical process is actually in control in the concentration range of the patients' samples.

d. The size of the analytical error is small relative to the requirements for medical usefulness. In this case, professional judgment is required, based on knowledge of the medical usefulness limits of errors (e.g., total error specifications), an understanding of the use and interpretation of the analytical results, and experience. The decision is best made in consultation with other experienced analysts or in consultation with the analyst's supervisor.

Example Interpretations of Control Data

Figure 4-5 shows some control measurements that could be obtained by applying the multi-rule procedure. The two control charts are for two different control materials analyzed in the same runs. The control values have been chosen to illustrate how the control rules should be interpreted in many different situations.

Run 5. The control measurement on the high-concentration material is within its 2s control limits, but the control measurement on the low-concentration material exceeds its −3s control limit. The analytical run should be rejected, based on a 1_{3s} rule violation. A random error has probably occurred.

Run 6. The control measurement on the high-concentration material exceeds its +2s limit, but the measurement on the low-concentration material is within its ±2s limits. This is a warning of a possible problem. Further inspection of the control data by using the 1_{3s}, 2_{2s}, and R_{4s} control rules does not confirm a problem. Application of the 4_{1s} and $10_{\bar{x}}$ control rules is not possible because the previous run was rejected and only the two control measurements in the current run are available. The run should be accepted.

Run 8. The control measurements on both materials exceed their respective +2s control limits; therefore, the run should be rejected, based on the 2_{2s} rule (applied across control materials). A systematic error has probably occurred throughout the concentration range covered by the control materials.

Run 11. The control measurements on both materials exceed their 2s control limits, but in opposite directions. The run should be rejected by the R_{4s} rule. A random error has probably occurred.

Run 13. The control measurement on the high-concentration material exceeds its −2s control limit, but the measurement on the low-

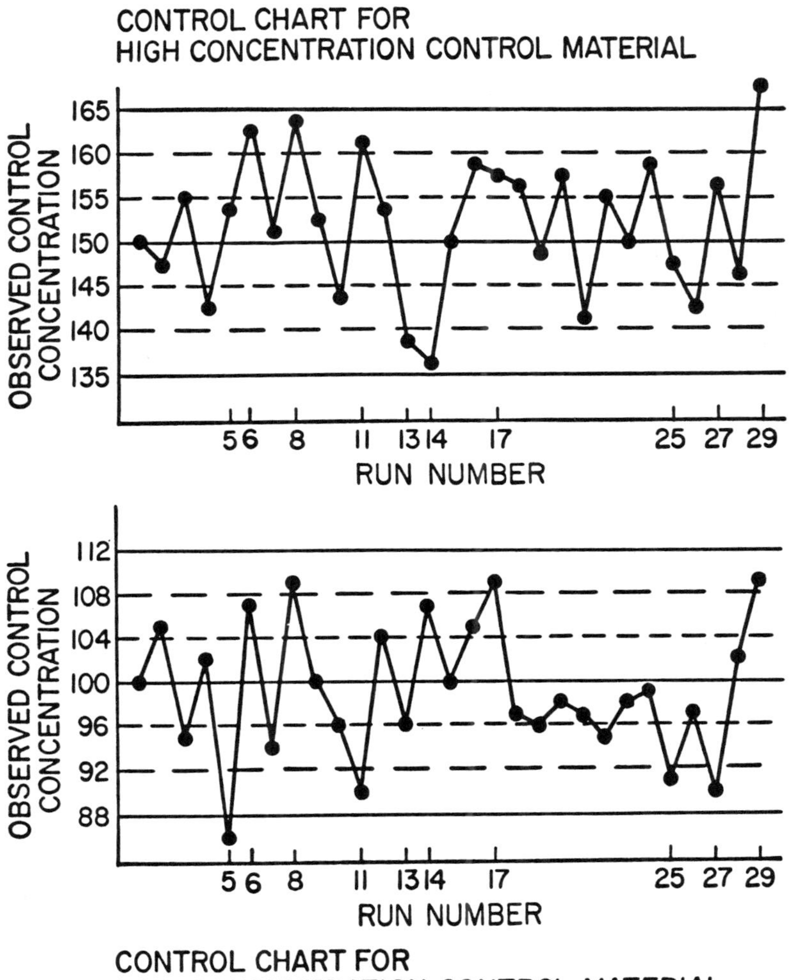

Fig. 4-5. Example of control charts for implementing a $1_{3s}/2_{2s}/R_{4s}/4_{1s}/10_{\bar{x}}$ multi-rule control procedure

The *top* chart is for a high-concentration control material and the *bottom* chart for a low-concentration control material. See text for interpretation. From Westgard et al. (7), reprinted with permission

concentration material is within 2s limits. This is a warning of a possible problem. Further inspection of the control data with use of the 1_{3s}, 2_{2s}, R_{4s}, and 4_{1s} control rule does not confirm a problem. Application of the $10_{\bar{x}}$ rule is not possible because run 11 was rejected and only four control measurements are available. The run should be accepted.

Run 14. The control measurement on the high-concentration material again exceeds its −2s control limit. The run should be rejected, based on the 2_{2s} control rule (applied within the high control, but across runs). A systematic error has probably occurred in the high concentration range.

Run 17. The control measurement on the low-concentration material exceeds its +2s control limit. The warning of a possible problem is confirmed, based on the 4_{1s} rule across materials. The last two measurements on each material exceed their respective +1s control limits, giving a total of four consecutive measurements exceeding +1s limits. The run should be rejected. A systematic error has probably occurred throughout the concentration range covered by the control materials.

Run 25. The control measurement on the low control exceeds its −2s control limit. Inspection by the other control rules does not provide ground for rejection. The run should be accepted.

Run 27. The control measurement on the low control exceeds its −2s control limit. Inspection reveals that the last 10 measurements on that material have fallen below the mean. The run should be rejected based on the $10_{\bar{x}}$ control rule. A systematic error has probably occurred.

Run 29. The control measurement on the high control exceeds its +3s control limit, and the control measurement on the low control exceeds its +2s control limit. The run can be rejected on the basis of either the 1_{3s} or 2_{2s} control rule. A systematic error has probably occurred throughout the concentration range covered by the control materials because both materials are exceeding their respective +2s control limits.

Alternative representations. Figure 4-6 shows how the same control data would appear when entered on tabular charts for each of the two control materials. Figure 4-7 shows the data on a *z*-score chart, which combines the measurements for the two control materials on a single chart.

Resolving Control Problems

When the multi-rule control procedure gives a rejection signal, a problem-solving process should be initiated. The first response by an analyst is often to prepare and re-analyze new samples of the control materials. However, this may not be the most productive response when the multi-rule control procedure is being used because (*a*) the number of false rejections should be low due to the choice of control rules, and (*b*) problems with the instability of the control materials themselves should have been reduced by including two different materials. Investigation of the measurement procedure itself may be more productive.

As a starting point, the particular control rule violated may indicate the type of error—random or systematic—that is occurring. Violation

High Concentration Control Material | **Low Concentration Control Material**

RUN #	High <−3s	High −3s	High −2s	High −1s	High $\bar{x}$	High +1s	High +2s	High +3s	High >+3s	Low <−3s	Low −3s	Low −2s	Low −1s	Low $\bar{x}$	Low +1s	Low +2s	Low +3s	Low >+3s	ACCEPT or REJECT	RULE VIOLATION
	≤134	135–139	140–144	145–149	150	151–155	156–160	161–165	≥166	≤87	88–91	92–95	96–99	100	101–104	105–108	109–112	≥113		
1					150									100					ACCEPT	
2				147												105			ACCEPT	
3						155						95							ACCEPT	
4			143												102				ACCEPT	
5						154				86									REJECT	1_{3S}
6								163								107			ACCEPT	1_{2S} WARNING ONLY
7						151						94							ACCEPT	
8								164									109		REJECT	2_{2S}
9						153								100					ACCEPT	
10			144										96						ACCEPT	
11								161			90								REJECT	R_{4S}
12						154									104				ACCEPT	
13		139											96						ACCEPT	1_{2S} WARNING ONLY
14		136														107			REJECT	2_{2S}
15					150									100					ACCEPT	
16							159									105			ACCEPT	
17							157										109		REJECT	4_{1S}
18							156						97						ACCEPT	
19				149									96						ACCEPT	
20							157						98						ACCEPT	
21			141										97						ACCEPT	
22						155						95							ACCEPT	
23					150								98						ACCEPT	
24							159						99						ACCEPT	
25				147							91								ACCEPT	1_{2S} WARNING ONLY
26			142										97						ACCEPT	
27							156				90								REJECT	$10_{\bar{x}}$
28				146											102				ACCEPT	
29									167								109		REJECT	1_{3S} AND 2_{2S}

Fig. 4-6. Example application with two tabular charts for implementing a $1_{3s}/2_{2s}/R_{4s}/4_{1s}/10_{\bar{x}}$ multi-rule control procedure

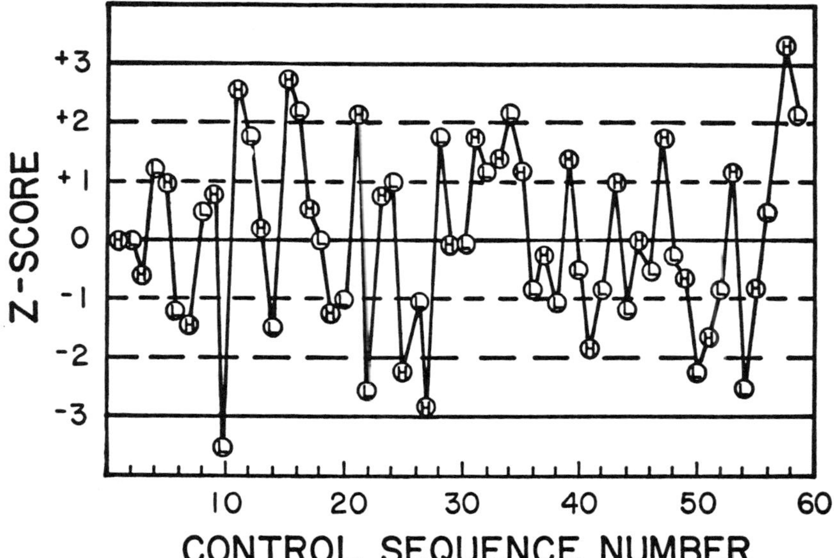

Fig. 4-7. Example application of a single z-score chart for implementing a $1_{3s}/2_{2s}/R_{4s}/4_{1s}/10_{\bar{x}}$ multi-rule control procedure

Control measurements for the high-concentration material are indicated by *H* and those for the low-concentration material by *L*

of the 2_{2s}, 4_{1s}, or $10_{\bar{x}}$ rules suggests a systematic error, whereas violation of the 1_{3s} or R_{4s} rules suggests a random error. When systematic errors are large, 1_{3s} violations will also be observed, in addition to the violations noted previously; when random errors are large, any control rule may be violated. The rule violated is not an absolute indicator of the type of error occurring, but it suggests the first direction for investigation of the problem.

The type of error occurring is important because it in turn suggests possible causes or sources of the problem. For example, violation of the 2_{2s} control rule in run 8 (Figure 4-5) suggests a systematic error throughout the concentration range tested by the two control materials. When the violation occurs on two different control materials within the run, it is unlikely to be a problem with the control materials themselves. It is more likely a problem with the calibrator solutions, instrument calibration, reagent blanks, or similar factors that will affect all of the measurements in the same direction.

When a random error occurs, such as suggested by violation of the R_{4s} rule on run 11 (Figure 4-5), several different causes are suggested: instability of the reagents or measurement conditions; variability in timing, pipetting, or individual technique; or other similar factors. The possible sources of errors depend on the particular measurement procedure and the nature of the reagents and instruments used. The analyst will be assisted by the manufacturer's troubleshooting guidelines, documentation of reagent and instrument changes, documentation of previous problems, and experience.

When a control problem has been resolved, there remains a question of what should be done with the control data from the out-of-control run; should they be included in further assessment of control status and in further data calculations? In assessing control status after using problem-solving procedures, the analyst's objective should be to assess control of the newly corrected measurement procedure. This is best done by increasing the number of control measurements in that next run, rather than utilizing any measurements from a previous run. In performing calculations with control data to update the control limits, the purpose is to characterize only the stable performance of the measurement procedure. Data obtained during unstable operation (out-of-control situations) should not be included because it increases s, which widens the control limits and reduces the error-detection capabilities of the control procedure.

Performance Characteristics

The detection of both intermittent and persistent errors should be considered, which requires that probabilities for rejection and average run lengths be determined. The evaluation of performance is somewhat more complicated than for single-rule procedures, because this multirule procedure effectively accumulates past control measurements by the inclusion of the 4_{1s} and $10_{\bar{x}}$ control rules.

Probabilities for rejection. Power-function graphs are given in Figures 4-8 and 4-9. The detection of random error is shown by the power curves in Figure 4-8, the different curves being for different numbers of control measurements per run. No additional detection of random error is gained from use of past control data because the 1_{3s} and R_{4s} rules are applied only within a single run (to maintain their selectivity to random rather than systematic errors).

The upper left panel of Figure 4-9 describes the probabilities for detecting systematic errors when N = 2. The different power curves correspond to different numbers of runs (r), each with N = 2, and illustrate how the error detection increases from run to run when the analytical errors persist. The increase in error detection comes from the use of control rules across runs, thereby increasing the effective number of control measurements from two (r = 1) to four (r = 2) to 10 (r = 5). The 4_{1s} rule can be applied after two runs have been accumulated, the $10_{\bar{x}}$ rule after five runs.

When N = 4, the detection of systematic errors is described in the

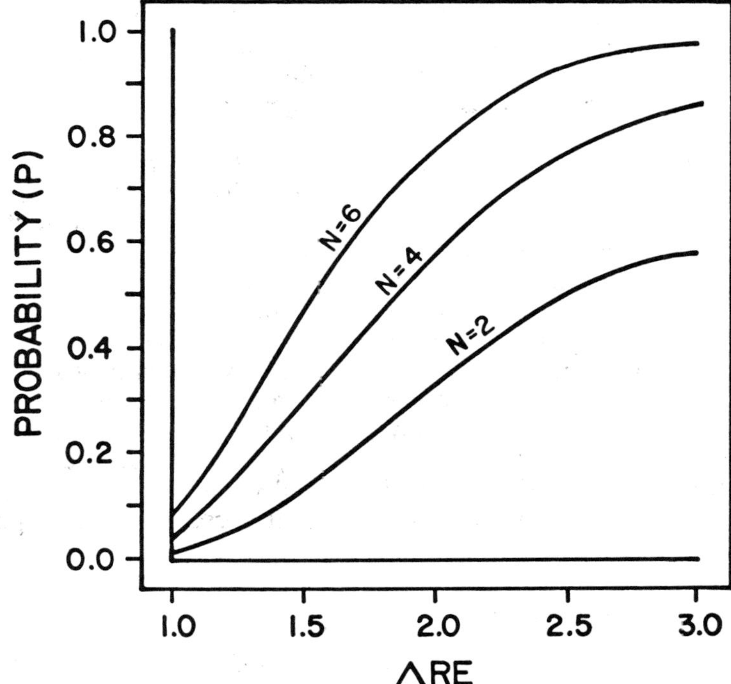

Fig. 4-8. Power-function graph for a $1_{3s}/2_{2s}/R_{4s}/4_{1s}/10_{\bar{x}}$ multi-rule control procedure for detecting random error with N = 2, 4, and 6

upper right panel of Figure 4-9. The 4_{1s} rule is used for all individual runs, but the $10_{\bar{x}}$ rule is used only when errors persist for three runs or more.

When N = 6, the detection of systematic errors is described in the lower left panel of Figure 4-9. The lower curve shows the power attained in a single run and the upper curve shows the power after two runs. Note that the probability of false rejections increases, limiting this multi-rule algorithm to $N \leq 6$.

Average run lengths. The calculation procedures outlined in Chapter 3 are used for determining the average run lengths from the probabilities for rejection given in the power-function graphs above. The average run length for acceptable quality (ARL_a) can be calculated from the probability for false rejection by use of equation 3-1 ($ARL_a = 1/P_{fr}$). The average run length for rejectable quality (ARL_r) requires use of equation 3-2 and the tabular calculation procedure because the probability for error detection is not constant from run to run as it was in the earlier example (Table 3-4). The changing value of P_{ed} is taken into account by using the probability appropriate for the run number.

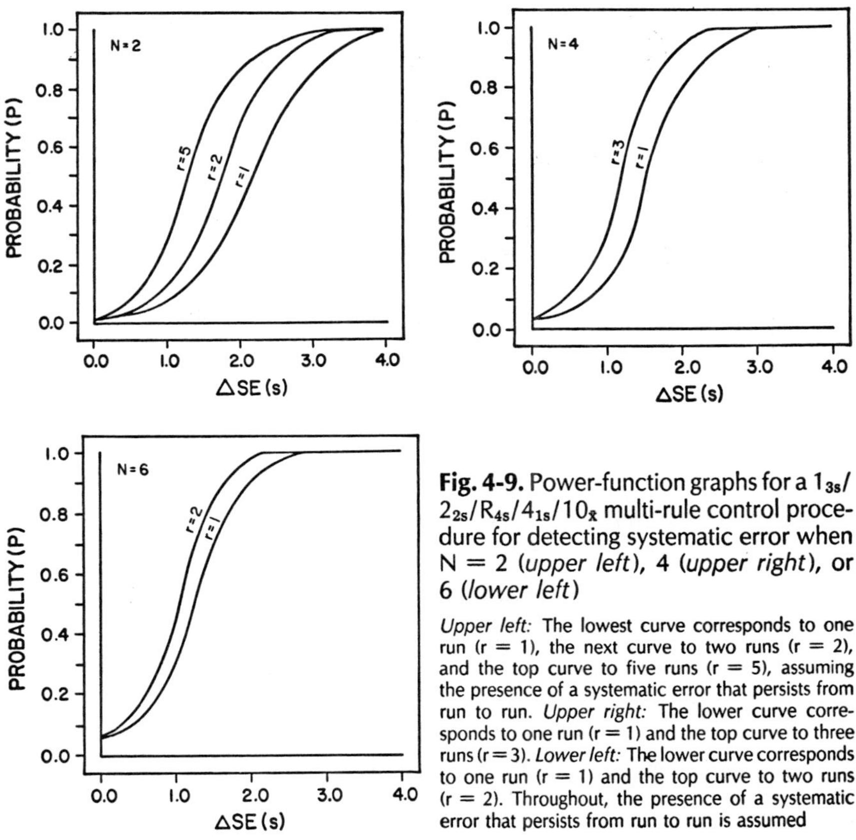

Fig. 4-9. Power-function graphs for a $1_{3s}/2_{2s}/R_{4s}/4_{1s}/10_{\bar{x}}$ multi-rule control procedure for detecting systematic error when N = 2 (*upper left*), 4 (*upper right*), or 6 (*lower left*)

Upper left: The lowest curve corresponds to one run (r = 1), the next curve to two runs (r = 2), and the top curve to five runs (r = 5), assuming the presence of a systematic error that persists from run to run. *Upper right:* The lower curve corresponds to one run (r = 1) and the top curve to three runs (r = 3). *Lower left:* The lower curve corresponds to one run (r = 1) and the top curve to two runs (r = 2). Throughout, the presence of a systematic error that persists from run to run is assumed

Table 4-1 shows an example calculation of ARL_r for the $1_{3s}/2_{2s}/R_{4s}/4_{1s}/10_{\bar{x}}$ multi-rule control procedure for detection of a persistent systematic shift equivalent to 1.5s. The probabilities for error detection are obtained from the power-function graph in Figure 4-8, which shows a probability of 0.19 for detecting a 1.5s shift in the first run in which it occurs, 0.36 when the error persists for two to four runs, and 0.66 when the error persists for five or more runs. Note in Table 4-1 that the probability of 0.19 is entered for run number 1, 0.36 for runs 2 through 4, and 0.66 for runs 5 and higher. The average run length is calculated to be 2.98, meaning that it would take about three runs, on the average, before a persistent shift equivalent to a 1.5s would be detected.

Average run lengths should be determined for errors of different sizes. Table 4-2 provides a summary for the $1_{3s}/2_{2s}/R_{4s}/4_{1s}/10_{\bar{x}}$ multi-rule control procedure described above. The average run length for

Table 4-1. Calculation of Average Run Length (ARL) for the $1_{3s}/2_{2s}/R_{4s}/4_{1s}/10_{\bar{x}}$ Multi-Rule Control Procedure: N = 2, Systematic Shift Equivalent to 1.5s

Run no. (or run length)	P_{ed}, this run	Proportion of errors: Undetected before this run	Detected this run	Cumulative detected	Calculated contribution to ARL
1	0.190	1.000	0.190	0.190	0.190
2	0.360	0.810	0.292	0.482	0.583
3	0.360	0.518	0.187	0.668	0.560
4	0.360	0.332	0.119	0.788	0.478
5	0.660	0.212	0.140	0.928	0.701
6	0.660	0.072	0.048	0.975	0.286
7	0.660	0.025	0.016	0.992	0.113
8	0.660	0.008	0.006	0.997	0.044
9	0.660	0.003	0.002	0.999	0.017
10	0.660	0.001	0.001	1.000	0.006
11	0.660	0.000	0.000	1.000	0.002
12	0.660	0.000	0.000	1.000	0.001
					ARL = 2.982

an error of 0.0s corresponds to the average run length between false rejections (ARL_a). The other figures indicate the average run lengths for systematic errors from 0.5s to 3.0s (ARL_r). Similar calculations could be made for increases in random error, but because P_{ed} does not change from run to run for this particular multi-rule procedure, ARL_r for persistent random errors can be estimated simply as $1/P_{ed}$.

Example application: urea nitrogen. To compare the performance of the $1_{3s}/2_{2s}/R_{4s}/4_{1s}/10_{\bar{x}}$ multi-rule procedure with that of Levey–Jennings charts, we will again use the urea nitrogen example from Chapter 2, where the critical sizes of medically important errors were calculated

Table 4-2. Average Run Lengths for the $1_{3s}/2_{2s}/R_{4s}/4_{1s}/10_{\bar{x}}$ Multi-Rule Control Procedure with N = 2 for Different Sizes of Systematic Errors

Size of systematic shift	Average run length
0.0s	100
0.5s	19
1.0s	5.9
1.5s	3.0
2.0s	2.0
3.0s	1.2

Table 4-3. Average Run Length (ARL) Calculations for the $1_{3s}/2_{2s}/R_{4s}/4_{1s}/10_{\bar{x}}$ Multi-Rule Control Procedure: Systematic Shift Equivalent to 1.83s

Run no. (or run length)	P_{ed}, this run	Proportion of errors: Undetected before this run	Detected this run	Cumulative detected	Calculated contribution to ARL
N = 2					
1	0.330	1.000	0.330	0.330	0.330
2	0.550	0.670	0.369	0.699	0.737
3	0.550	0.301	0.166	0.864	0.497
4	0.550	0.136	0.075	0.939	0.298
5	0.820	0.061	0.050	0.989	0.250
6	0.820	0.011	0.009	0.998	0.054
7	0.820	0.002	0.002	1.000	0.011
8	0.820	0.000	0.000	1.000	0.002
9	0.820	0.000	0.000	1.000	0.000
10	0.820	0.000	0.000	1.000	0.000
					ARL = 2.182
N = 4					
1	0.740	1.000	0.740	0.740	0.740
2	0.740	0.260	0.192	0.932	0.385
3	0.900	0.068	0.061	0.993	0.183
4	0.900	0.007	0.006	0.999	0.024
5	0.900	0.001	0.001	1.000	0.003
					ARL = 1.335

as $\Delta RE_c = 1.78$ and $\Delta SE_c = 1.83s$. From Figure 4-8, the probabilities for false rejection are 0.01 for N = 2 and 0.03 for N = 4, corresponding to ARL_a values of 100 (1/0.01) and 33 (1/0.03), respectively. The probabilities for detecting the critical random error are 0.24 when N = 2 and 0.47 when N = 4. Because no additional error detection is gained from use of past control data, P_{ed} is constant and the ARL_r for the critical random error can be calculated as $1/P_{ed}$, giving values of 4.2 (1/0.24) and 2.1 (1/0.47).

From Figure 4-9, the probabilities for detecting the critical systematic error when N = 2 are 0.33 for an intermittent error that occurs in an individual run (r = 1 curve, upper left panel), 0.55 when the error persists for two runs (r = 2 curve), and 0.82 when the error persists for five runs (r = 5 curve). ARL_r is calculated as 2.18, as shown in Table 4-3. When N = 4, the probabilities for detecting the critical systematic error are 0.74 in the first run (r = 1 curve, upper right

Table 4-4. Performance of the $1_{3s}/2_{2s}/R_{4s}/4_{1s}/10_{\bar{x}}$ Multi-Rule Control Procedure and Levey–Jennings Charts Compared

Control procedure	N	No error P_{fr}	No error ARL_a	$\Delta RE_c = 1.78$ P_{ed}	$\Delta RE_c = 1.78$ ARL_r	$\Delta SE_c = 1.83s$ P_{ed}	$\Delta SE_c = 1.83s$ ARL_r
1_{2s}	1	0.05	20	0.26	3.8	0.42	2.4
	2	0.10	10	0.43	2.3	0.67	1.5
	4	0.18	5.6	0.75	1.3	0.90	1.1
1_{3s}	1	0.01	100	0.07	14	0.10	10
	2	0.01	100	0.14	7.1	0.17	5.9
	4	0.01	100	0.33	3.0	0.38	2.6
	8	0.02	50	0.51	2.0	0.57	1.8
Multi-rule	2	0.01	100	0.24	4.2	0.33	2.2
	4	0.03	33	0.47	2.1	0.74	1.3

panel) and 0.90 when the error persists for three runs (r = 3 curve). ARL_r is calculated as 1.33.

The performances of Levey–Jennings charts are compared with that of the $1_{3s}/2_{2s}/R_{4s}/4_{1s}/10_{\bar{x}}$ multi-rule procedure in Table 4-4. In comparison with Levey–Jennings charts with ±2s control limits (1_{2s} rule), the multi-rule procedure with N = 2 provides nearly the same error detection as 1_{2s} with N = 1; the multi-rule procedure with N = 4 provides about the same error detection as 1_{2s} with N = 2. In both cases, the multi-rule procedure will cause fewer false rejections. The same quality can be assured without the loss in productivity from the greater number of false rejections of the 1_{2s} procedure, although the gain in productivity would be offset somewhat by the increase in the number of control measurements.

In comparison with the Levey–Jennings chart with ±3s limits, when N = 2, the multi-rule procedure detects nearly twice as many errors, with little or no change in the rate of false rejections. Improved quality is achieved without any increase in the number of control measurements because the control measurements are being more critically interpreted. When N = 4, the error detection of the multi-rule procedure is again much better than that for the 1_{3s} procedure, especially for systematic errors, both intermittent and persistent. Use of the multi-rule procedure thus would improve the quality of the analytical process with little effect on productivity. In fact, the multi-rule procedure with N = 4 performs nearly the same as a 1_{3s} control procedure with N = 8. Thus, use of the multi-rule procedure will provide about the same quality, but with improved productivity because fewer control measurements would be required.

Table 4-5. Average Run Lengths for the $1_{2.5s}$ Single-Rule and the $1_{3s}/2_{2s}/R_{4s}/4_{1s}/10_{\bar{x}}$ Multi-Rule Control Procedures (N = 2)

Size of systematic shift	Average run lengths	
	$1_{2.5s}$	$1_{3s}/2_{2s}/R_{4s}/4_{1s}/10_{\bar{x}}$
0.0s	36	100
0.5s	29	19
1.0s	8.1	5.9
1.5s	3.3	3.0
2.0s	1.9	2.0
3.0s	1.1	1.2

Example application: comparison with a $1_{2.5s}$ procedure. Blum (*4*) has suggested that a $1_{2.5s}$ single-rule procedure has the same performance as the $1_{3s}/2_{2s}/R_{4s}/4_{1s}/10_{\bar{x}}$ multi-rule procedure. For N = 2 and the detection of intermittent errors, the probabilities for error detection for a $1_{2.5s}$ control procedure are similar (see the power-function graphs for the $1_{2.5s}$ rule in Appendix II) because only the two control measurements within a run are used and only the 1_{3s}, 2_{2s}, and R_{4s} rules can be used. For N = 2 and persistent systematic errors, the 4_{1s} and $10_{\bar{x}}$ control rules can be applied, increasing the error detection of the multi-rule procedure. The average run lengths of the two procedures are compared in Table 4-5. The $1_{3s}/2_{2s}/R_{4s}/4_{1s}/10_{\bar{x}}$ multi-rule generally has a better (longer) ARL_a, 100 vs 36; better (shorter) ARL_r values for systematic shifts in the range 0.5s to 1.5s; and nearly equivalent ARL_r values for large systematic errors.

Other Multi-Rule Control Procedures

Modified Westgard Multi-Rule Procedures

The $1_{3s}/2_{2s}/R_{4s}/4_{1s}/10_{\bar{x}}$ algorithm discussed above provides a generally useful control procedure, but its practicality and performance may be improved in certain situations. The control rules may be changed; in certain cases, some may even be eliminated. Other control rules may be more suitable for a specified number of control measurements. And some rules may be better interpreted as "warning" rather than "rejection" signals.

Modifications for computer implementation. The 1_{2s} rule is recommended as a warning rule for manual implementations to minimize the time required for data inspections. A careful assessment of control status is very important when a 1_{2s} rule violation warns of possible problems. When there is no warning, looking back through control measurements to test the 4_{1s} and $10_{\bar{x}}$ rules may take too much time; therefore, application of those rules need not be required in a manual implementation. In principle, 4_{1s} and $10_{\bar{x}}$ violations could occur without ever causing a 1_{2s} warning, but simulation studies have shown no differences between the power-function graphs for 1_{2s}-triggered application of the rules and automatic application of all the rules.

When the multi-rule procedure is implemented via computer, the 1_{2s} rule may be eliminated and the other rules tested automatically. There is no need for the 1_{2s} warning because the computer can easily check the data for conformance with all the rules.

Modifications for different values of N. When N changes, one should consider the use of different rules. When N = 1, the algorithm can be reduced to a 1_{2s} control rule for run rejection. For N = 2 or 4, all of the rules can be used, for maximum error detection. Some can be applied within a run and some can be applied across runs, making use of data from past runs to increase the detection of systematic errors that persist from run to run. Table 4-6 summarizes what rules might be used as N changes.

For N = 3, the rule $(2 \text{ of } 3)_{2s}$ can be used to reject a run when two out of three measurements exceed a given 2s control limit (*8*); note that the rule does not require two consecutive measurements to exceed a 2s limit, only two out of the last three. The use of a 3_{1s} rule instead of a 4_{1s} rule is not recommended because the false rejections are likely to increase, especially for measurement procedures where substantial run-to-run changes (large between-run standard deviation, s_b) have not been eliminated during the optimization of the measurement procedure.

A $12_{\bar{x}}$ rule is more generally useful than a $10_{\bar{x}}$ rule because it more easily fits with runs having two, three, four, or six control measure-

Table 4-6. Summary of Control Rules Appropriate for Different Numbers of Control Measurements

N	Recommended control rules: Individual runs	Consecutive runs
1	1_{2s}	4_{1s}
2	$1_{3s}/2_{2s}/R_{4s}$	$4_{1s}/10_{\bar{x}}$ or $12_{\bar{x}}$
3	$1_{3s}/(2 \text{ of } 3)_{2s}/R_{4s}$	$9_{\bar{x}}$ or $12_{\bar{x}}$
4	$1_{3s}/2_{2s}/R_{4s}/4_{1s}$	$8_{\bar{x}}$ or $12_{\bar{x}}$
6	$1_{3s}/2_{2s}/R_{0.01}/4_{1s}$	$12_{\bar{x}}$

ments. For example, when N = 3, it makes little sense to use a $10_{\bar{x}}$ rule and look back three and one-third runs; use either a $9_{\bar{x}}$ rule and look back three runs, or a $12_{\bar{x}}$ rule and look back four runs. Likewise for N = 4, it is better to use either an $8_{\bar{x}}$ rule and look back two runs, or a $12_{\bar{x}}$ rule and look back three runs.

For higher values of N, Carey et al. (*9,10*) have investigated different rules, e.g., rules of the type m of n outside of k standard deviations, either one- or two-sided. Simulation programs having generic rules of these types should prove useful in optimizing the design of multi-rule procedures for higher values of N. Also consider the use of mean and range procedures, or mean and standard deviation charts (or chi-square rules).

Modifications to reduce false rejections. When N = 6, the false-rejection rate will increase, mainly because of false rejections from the R_{4s} rule. Elimination of the R_{4s} rule will reduce the number of false rejections without affecting the detection of systematic errors, but will decrease the detection of random errors. Modifying the R_{4s} rule by increasing the control limits to 4.8s will keep the false rejections suitably low while maintaining reasonable detection of random errors. In effect, this amounts to implementing a quantitative range procedure, a $R_{0.01}$ control rule, while maintaining the other control rules for detection of systematic errors (see factors for control limits in Appendix I, Table AI-2; e.g., for N = 6, the factor is 4.76).

Modifications to reduce error detection. Analysts should recognize that the 4_{1s} and $10_{\bar{x}}$ rules are sensitive to small systematic errors, which, in some situations, may not be considered large enough to require rejection of an analytical run. For example, some instrument systems may show small shifts related to lot-to-lot differences in reagents. If re-calibrating the instrument fails to eliminate small lot-to-lot shifts, the 4_{1s} and $10_{\bar{x}}$ rules will continue to detect the shifts and repeatedly alert the analyst to their presence—which has already been made known. If it is determined that the shifts cannot be further reduced or corrected, then the continuing rejection signals become an annoyance. In such cases, the use of the rules should be discontinued once a judgment is made that the shifts can not be further reduced or eliminated. Otherwise, they have the same effect as "false alarms" and may compromise future responses when additional problems occur.

Modifications to use for warning purposes. Instead of eliminating the 4_{1s} and $10_{\bar{x}}$ rules, one can interpret them as warning rules to trigger inspection of the measurement procedure before undertaking new analytical runs, or to invoke maintenance procedures to prevent errors from getting large enough to cause run rejection. Figure 4-10 diagrams the logic for using a multi-rule procedure involving the 4_{1s} and $10_{\bar{x}}$ rules to trigger preventive maintenance procedures.

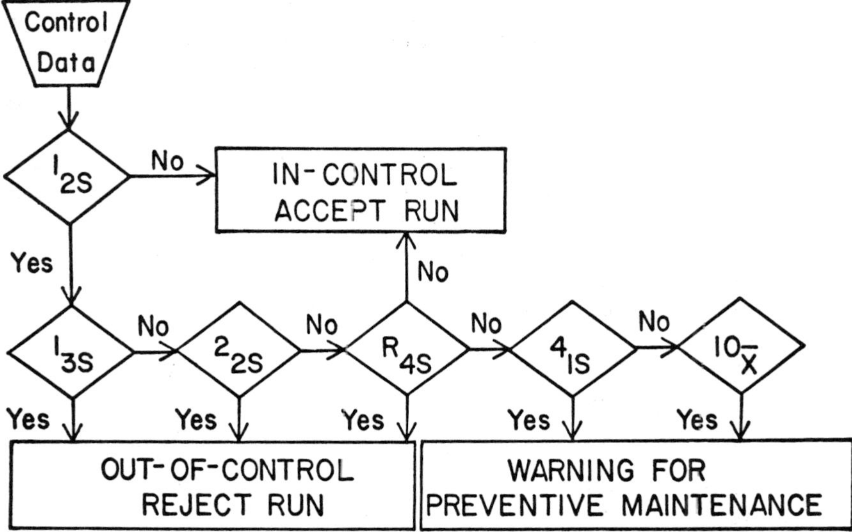

Fig. 4-10. Logic diagram for a modified $1_{3s}/2_{2s}/R_{4s}/4_{1s}/10_{\bar{x}}$ multi-rule control procedure in which the 4_{1s} and $10_{\bar{x}}$ rules provide "warnings" for preventive maintenance procedures

Blum Multi-Rule Procedure

Blum has recommended a complex 10-rule procedure requiring computer implementation (*4*). The rules explicitly define retrospective data checking, including the use of range-type rules retrospectively across runs and materials. The performance of the Blum procedure has been characterized by computer simulation studies that assume that the analytical errors persist from run to run. However, the performance characteristics are not presented in terms of average run lengths, thus making interpretation of the results difficult. The performances of the Blum and Westgard multi-rule procedures appear to be similar for systematic error, but the Blum procedure should provide better detection of random error because data from past runs are used; however, that apparent gain could be offset by difficulties in distinguishing random errors and systematic errors.[1]

[1] The complexity of Blum's procedure and the increased difficulty in distinguishing the types of errors occurring make the procedure more difficult for laboratory analysts to use. It is not sufficient that a computer can do the calculations and interpretations: the laboratory analysts must understand what is being done. One of the objectives of quality control is to provide a basis for building a system for quality management, with the ultimate objective of developing the problem-solving skills that make error prevention a reality. Accomplishing this requires control techniques that strengthen the analyst's abilities to diagnose problems. The analyst must be able to understand what the control techniques are doing, even though a computer may be used to implement the procedures.

Implications for the Selection or Design of Control Procedures

For intermittent errors, the probability for rejection depends on the number of control measurements in a single run and the control rules used to test that single run. In general, when N is 1 to 4, control rules such as 1_{2s} or 1_{3s} can be used to test the tails of the error distribution. Moving the control limits closer to the mean of the distribution will increase error detection, but will also increase false rejections.

Although a single-rule control procedure may be satisfactory for detecting intermittent errors, the detection of persistent errors can always be improved by adding another control rule. The example given in Table 4-7 illustrates this point, using average run lengths to compare the performance of the different designs. Because the detection of persistent errors can always be improved by making a single-rule procedure into a multi-rule procedure, Blum's recommendation (*4*) for single-rule procedures with control limits from 2.3s to 2.6s should be regarded with some caution.

For persistent errors, additional control rules can be selected to test control measurements as they accumulate. With each additional run (up to the third, fourth, or fifth runs), one can add another control rule to test the control data. An example would be the use of the $1_{2.5s}$ rule for two control measurements in a run, addition of the 4_{1s} control rule to test the four measurements available after two runs, and addition of a $(5 \text{ of } 6)_{0.5s}$ rule to test the six control measurements available after three runs. Average run lengths need to be determined to evaluate a specific design and to compare different designs.

From this structuring of the control procedure to make use of the accumulated control measurements, the transition from a multi-rule procedure to a cusum procedure would be expected as a logical pro-

Table 4-7. Average Run Lengths for the $1_{2.5s}$ Single-Rule Control Procedure and for Multi-Rule Procedures That Include the $1_{2.5s}$ Rule (N = 2)

Size of systematic shift	Control rules			
	$1_{2.5s}$	$1_{2.5s}/4_{1s}$	$1_{2.5s}/4_{1s}/(5 \text{ of } 6)_{0.5s}$	$1_{2.5s}/4_{1s}/8_{\bar{x}}$
0.0s	36	34	22	27
0.5s	29	17	7.5	9.8
1.0s	8.1	6.5	3.4	4.2
1.5s	3.3	2.5	2.2	2.4
2.0s	1.9	1.6	1.6	1.6
3.0s	1.1	1.1	1.1	1.1

gression. Control rules such as 4_{1s} and $10_{\bar{x}}$ consider the approximate distance of control measurements from the mean of the control material by counting how many measurements fall outside of certain limits. A cusum procedure considers the exact distance of each control measurement from a target value, usually the mean for the control material, adding that difference to the cumulative sum of previous distances. Although such a cusum procedure can be expected to provide maximum detection of systematic errors, it will not be very sensitive to random errors. A cusum rule should be coupled with another control rule to provide better detection of random errors, again supporting the selection of a multi-rule procedure. Multi-rule procedures that include cusum rules have been developed and are suitable for manual and computer applications (*3,5*).

Summary

When individual control measurements or values are to be analyzed to assess control status, use of multiple criteria or multiple control rules can improve the performance of the control procedure. "Multi-rule" control procedures are a logical progression after "single-rule" procedures such as Levey–Jennings charts. The false-rejection problem of the Levey–Jennings chart with 2s control limits can be reduced; the error detection can be improved over that of the Levey–Jennings chart having 3s control limits. All that is required is a more critical interpretation of the control data by use of multiple decision criteria.

Multi-rule procedures can be tailored to fit individual measurement procedures, and their unique characteristics and requirements, by the choice of the control rules and of the number of control measurements. Such tailoring and individualized designs are a natural evolution in the search for more optimal quality control. This search can be guided by careful evaluation of the performance of the different designs, with determinations of their probabilities for rejection and average run lengths under conditions that allow comparison with the performance characteristics of other control procedures.

References

1. Westgard JO, Barry PL, Hunt MR, Groth T. A multi-rule Shewhart chart for quality control in clinical chemistry. Clin Chem 1981;27:493–501.

2. Haven GT. Outline for quality control decisions. Pathologist 1974;28:373–8.

3. Westgard JO, Groth T, Aronsson T, de Verdier C-H. Combined Shewhart–cusum control chart for improved quality control in clinical chemistry. Clin Chem 1977;23:1881–7.

4. Blum AS. Computer evaluation of statistical procedures, and a new quality-control statistical procedure. Clin Chem 1985;31:206–12.

5. Schoen I, Custer E, Graham G, Bandi Z, Surovik MH. Quality control log with CUSUM and clinically useful limits criteria. Arch Pathol Lab Med 1985;109:333–9.

6. Nelson LS. The Shewhart control chart—tests for special causes. J Qual Technol 1984;16:237–9.

7. Nelson LS. Interpreting Shewhart $\bar{x}$ control charts. J Qual Technol 1985;17:114–7.

8. Westgard JO, Groth T. Design and evaluation of statistical control procedures: applications of a computer "Quality Control Simulator" program. Clin Chem 1981;27:1536–45.

9. Eckert GH, Carey RN. Application of statistical control rules to quality control in radioimmunoassay. J Clin Immunoassay 1985;8:107–11.

10. Carey RN, Tyvoll JL, Plaut DS, Hancock MS, Barry PL, Westgard JO. Performance characteristics of some statistical quality control rules for radioimmunoassay. J Clin Immunoassay 1985;8:245–52.

CHAPTER 5

Predicting the Quality of an Analytical Process

"Cost-effective quality control" is concerned with selecting or designing a control procedure to maximize both the quality and productivity of an analytical process. Both quality and productivity depend on the performance characteristics of the measurement and control procedures.

The critical performance characteristic of the measurement procedure is its frequency of medically important errors. When measurement procedures are stable and errors are few, quality and productivity will be high. The critical performance characteristics of the control procedure are its probabilities for error detection and false rejection (or average run lengths). When control procedures have high rates of error detection, any errors that occur will be detected, the affected analytical runs rejected, and high quality maintained. When control procedures have high rates of error detection and few false rejections, productivity will be high because there will be few repeat runs and few repeat assay requests.

Control procedures having both a high probability for error detection (or short run length for rejectable quality) and a low probability for false rejection (or long run length for acceptable quality) generally require many control measurements per run, even when sensitive multirule procedures are used. Such control procedures will be costly unless the analytical runs are very large. On the other hand, large runs themselves may be costly if they slow the reporting of test results and delay the diagnosis and treatment of patients.

Can control procedures be selected or designed to provide high quality without requiring too many control measurements? Do the requirements for high error detection and low false rejection change as the frequency of errors changes? Are there situations where high error detection can be attained without concern for maintaining a low rate of false rejections, or where a low false-rejection rate is more important than high error detection? To answer such questions, managers and analysts need to understand how the quality of an analytical process depends on the frequency of errors associated with the measurement procedure, as well as the error-detection and false-rejection characteristics of the control procedure.

In this chapter, we introduce additional characteristics to describe the correctness of "accept" and "reject" signals from a control procedure and to predict the quality (defect rate) of the analytical process. (Prediction of the productivity of an analytical process is considered in Chapter 6.) We will show quantitatively how these additional characteristics depend on the frequency of errors of the measurement procedure and the error-detection and false-rejection characteristics of the control procedure, then illustrate their meaning by making some calculations for the urea nitrogen example that was introduced earlier.

Predictive Value Characteristics of an Analytical Process

We use the phrase "predictive value characteristics" here to distinguish these new characteristics from the "performance characteristics" introduced earlier. Performance characteristics are primary features of the measurement and control procedures, describing their individual performance. Predictive value characteristics are secondary features, depending on the primary characteristics, but also describing their combined effects on the analytical process. The predictive value characteristics are important for understanding the interaction between the measurement and control procedures and for predicting how the resulting analytical process will behave.

In Chapter 3, analytical runs were classified in terms of true rejects (tr), false rejects (fr), false accepts (fa), and true accepts (ta) (see Table 3-1). Table 5-1 shows an expanded list of characteristics that can be calculated on the basis of this classification of analytical runs. The probabilities for error detection (P_{ed}) and false rejection (P_{fr}), as well as average run lengths for rejectable quality (ARL_r) and acceptable quality (ARL_a), all considered earlier, describe how often a rejection signal is obtained for analytical runs with and without errors, respectively. Here we introduce three other terms—PV_r, PV_a, and $PV_{r\&a}$—to describe the correctness of the control decisions, i.e., to quantify how often the reject and accept decisions are correct. PV, the abbreviation for "predictive value," emphasizes that these characteristics predict how the analytical process will perform. Finally, the "defect rate" is included to predict the quality that is expected from the analytical process.

Correctness of reject decisions. The predictive value of a reject signal (PV_r) is the portion of reject signals that are true rejects—the number of true rejects divided by the total number of rejects (true rejects plus false rejects), presented as a proportion or percentage. Ideally, PV_r should be 1.00 or 100%, meaning that any reject signal is a true reject. A low value, such as 0.30, means that only 30% of the reject signals

Table 5-1. Performance and Predictive Value Characteristics of an Analytical Process

Analytical run	Reject signal	Accept signal	Totals
With error	n_{tr}	n_{fa}	$n_{tr} + n_{fa}$
Without error	n_{fr}	n_{ta}	$n_{fr} + n_{ta}$
Totals	$n_{tr} + n_{fr}$	$n_{fa} + n_{ta}$	n_t

Error detection	$P_{ed} = n_{tr}/(n_{tr} + n_{fa})$
False rejection	$P_{fr} = n_{fr}/(n_{fr} + n_{ta})$
Correctness of rejects	$PV_r = n_{tr}/(n_{tr} + n_{fr})$
Correctness of accepts	$PV_a = n_{ta}/(n_{fa} + n_{ta})$
Correctness of both	$PV_{r\&a} = (n_{tr} + n_{ta})/n_t$
Quality	Defect rate $= n_{fa}/n_t$

are true rejects; i.e., if a reject signal occurred, there would be only a 30% chance that an analytical run really had errors.

Correctness of accept decisions. The predictive value of an accept signal (PV_a) indicates the portion of accept signals that are true accepts—the number of true accepts divided by the total number of accepts (true accepts plus false accepts), presented as a proportion or percentage. Ideally, PV_a should also be 1.00 or 100%, meaning that any accept signal is a true accept. A low value, such as 0.50, means that only 50% of the accept signals are true accepts: only half the time would an accept signal correctly indicate that an analytical run was without errors.

Correctness of both reject and accept decisions. The predictive value of both reject and accept decisions ($PV_{r\&a}$) indicates the portion of *all* control decisions that are correct. It is the number of true rejects plus true accepts divided by the total number of runs (true rejects plus false rejects plus false accepts plus true accepts), and can be presented as a proportion or percentage. Ideally, $PV_{r\&a}$ should be 1.00 or 100%. A value of 0.70 means that only 70% of the control decisions are correct decisions; the other 30% are incorrect.

Quality of the analytical process. The quality of the analytical process is inversely related to the defect rate, defined in Chapter 2 as the portion of test results having "medically important errors." The defect rate can be predicted by the portion of analytical runs with errors that will be reported—the number of falsely accepted runs divided by the total number of runs, presented as a proportion or percentage. Ideally, the defect rate should be 0.00 or 0%, indicating that no medically important errors are present in the reported test results. A value of 0.05 means that 5% of the runs or patients' test results have medically important errors present.

Estimation of Predictive Value Characteristics from Probabilities for Rejection

The predictive value terms would be easy to calculate if data were available on the number of runs that are true rejects, false rejects, false accepts, and true accepts. For example, for an analytical process that produces 100 runs, including two true reject runs, eight false reject runs, 10 false accept runs, and 80 true accept runs, PV_r is $2/(2 + 8) = 20\%$, PV_a is $80/(10 + 80) = 89\%$, $PV_{r\&a}$ is $(2 + 80)/(2 + 8 + 10 + 80) = 82\%$, and the defect rate is $10/100 = 10\%$.

Estimating these terms by experimental determination of the number of runs in each class would be difficult and time consuming. All reject signals would have to be carefully investigated to distinguish between true and false rejections, requiring additional efforts at times when an analytical process is nonfunctional and needs to be fixed. All accept signals would have to be investigated to determine which are false acceptances, requiring additional efforts at times when the process is apparently functioning properly.

A better approach would be to calculate the predictive value terms from the performance characteristics of the analytical process. The predictive value terms depend on the error-detection and false-rejection characteristics of the control procedure, and on the number of analytical runs having medically important errors, which is a characteristic of the measurement procedure. Because they depend on the characteristics of both the control and measurement procedures, the predictive value terms are thus characteristics of the analytical process as a whole.

Table 5-2 summarizes the equations for calculating the predictive value characteristics as functions of the probabilities for error detection (P_{ed}) and false rejection (P_{fr}) of a control procedure and of the frequency of errors (f) of a measurement procedure. [See the addendum to this chapter for derivation of these equations.] To assess the behavior of an analytical process, we can use these equations to calculate the predictive value terms for a variety of process characteristics (*1*).

Predictive value of a reject signal. Figure 5-1 (top) shows the predictive value of a reject signal as a function of frequency of errors, f. The *y*-axis is scaled from 0 to 100 to present the predictive value as a percentage. Frequency of errors is also presented as a percentage of runs and is plotted with *logarithmic* scaling on the *x*-axis for better resolution of low frequencies of error. The different curves correspond to different values for P_{ed} and P_{fr}. When f is low, the highest (best) PV_r is achieved

Table 5-2. Predictive Value Characteristics as Functions of the Probability for Error Detection (P_{ed}), Probability for False Rejection (P_{fr}), and Frequency of Errors (f)

Analytical runs	Reject signal	Accept signal
With errors	$n_{tr} = n_t f P_{ed}$	$n_{fa} = n_t f(1 - P_{ed})$
Without errors	$n_{fr} = n_t(1 - f)P_{fr}$	$n_{ta} = n_t(1 - f)(1 - P_{fr})$

$$PV_r = \frac{n_{tr}}{n_{tr} + n_{fr}} = \frac{fP_{ed}}{fP_{ed} + (1 - f)P_{fr}}$$

$$PV_a = \frac{n_{ta}}{n_{ta} + n_{fa}} = \frac{(1 - f)(1 - P_{fr})}{(1 - f)(1 - P_{fr}) + f(1 - P_{ed})}$$

$$PV_{r\&a} = \frac{n_{tr} + n_{ta}}{n_t} = fP_{ed} + (1 - f)(1 - P_{fr})$$

$$\text{Defect rate} = n_{fa}/n_t = f(1 - P_{ed})$$

when P_{fr} is lowest. P_{ed} has less impact, although PV_r does improve a little as P_{ed} increases. At high frequencies of errors, the PV_r is high, regardless of the characteristics of the control procedure.

For cost-effective operation when a measurement procedure is stable (i.e., when f is low and few analytical errors are occurring), the predictive value of a reject signal should be high. Otherwise, analysts will waste much time and effort responding to reject signals that are unrelated to analytical problems. The control procedure should be selected primarily to have a low probability for false rejection

Predictive value of an accept signal. Figure 5-1 (bottom) shows PV_a as a function of frequency of errors, f. For high frequencies of errors, PV_a depends almost entirely on P_{ed}, increasing as P_{ed} increases. Differences due to changes in P_{fr} (in the range of 0.00 to 0.05) would hardly be visible on the graph. At low frequencies of errors, most control procedures achieve high PV_a values.

For cost-effective operation when a measurement procedure is unstable (i.e., when f is high and there are many analytical errors), the predictive value of an accept signal should be high. Otherwise, patients' results will be reported even though errors may be present, causing physicians to request the tests again to obtain useful results. The control procedure should be selected primarily to have a high probability for error detection, with little concern for its probability for false rejection.

Predictive value of both reject and accept signals. Figure 5-2 is a plot of $PV_{r\&a}$ vs frequency of errors, with *linear* scaling on the x-axis. At low frequencies of errors, $PV_{r\&a}$ depends primarily on P_{fr}, whereas at high frequencies of error it depends primarily on P_{ed}. The relationship is

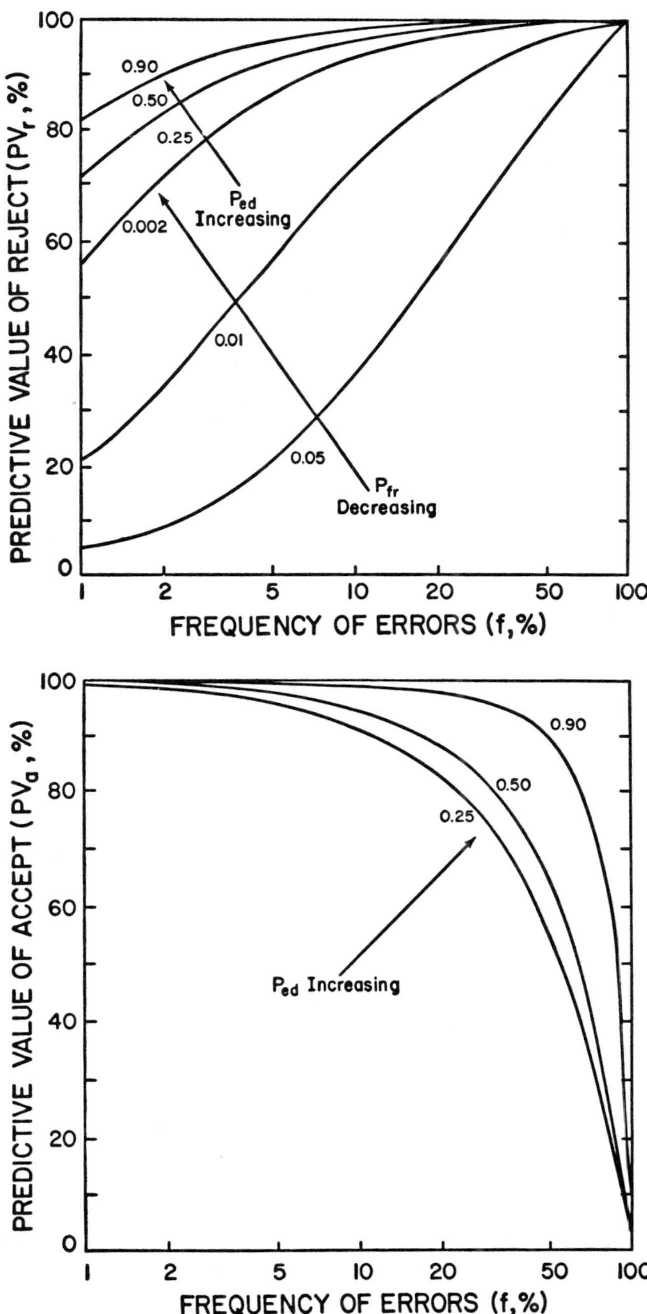

Fig. 5-1. Correctness of reject signals (*top*) and accept signals (*bottom*) as a function of the frequency of errors in the measurement procedure

The predictive value of a reject signal or of an accept signal (PV_r and PV_a, respectively) is plotted vs the frequency of errors (f). From Westgard and Groth (7), reprinted with permission

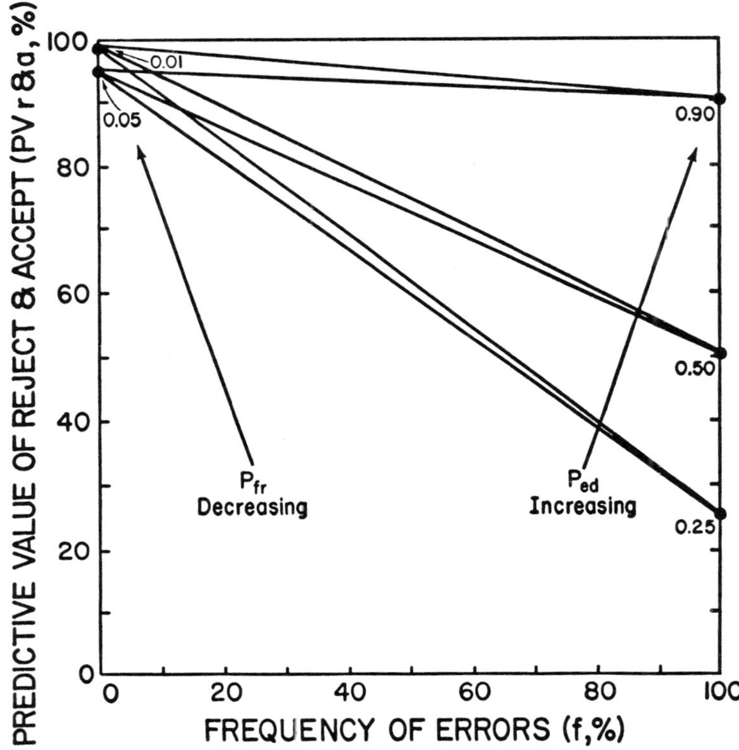

Fig. 5-2. Correctness of both reject and accept signals as a function of the frequency of errors in the measurement procedure

The predictive value of both reject and accept signals ($PV_{r\&a}$) is plotted vs the frequency of errors (f). From Westgard and Groth (7), reprinted with permission

linear and can be drawn from knowledge of P_{fr} and P_{ed} alone: plot $1 - P_{fr}$ for 0% frequency of errors and plot P_{ed} for 100% frequency of errors, then connect the two points by a straight line.

The plot of $PV_{r\&a}$ illustrates that the overall correctness of control signals depends on P_{ed} and P_{fr}, and points out that the characteristic of the control procedure that is most important depends on what frequency of errors is of interest. At low f, performance is determined primarily by P_{fr}. At high f, performance is determined primarily by P_{ed}. A perfect control procedure, having low P_{fr} and high P_{ed}, would perform well at either low or high frequencies of errors.

Defect rate. What defect rate to expect depends on the frequency of errors of the measurement procedure and the error detection capability of the control procedure, as shown in Figure 5-3. Increasing P_{ed} causes the defect rate to decrease. Changes in P_{fr} do not by themselves change

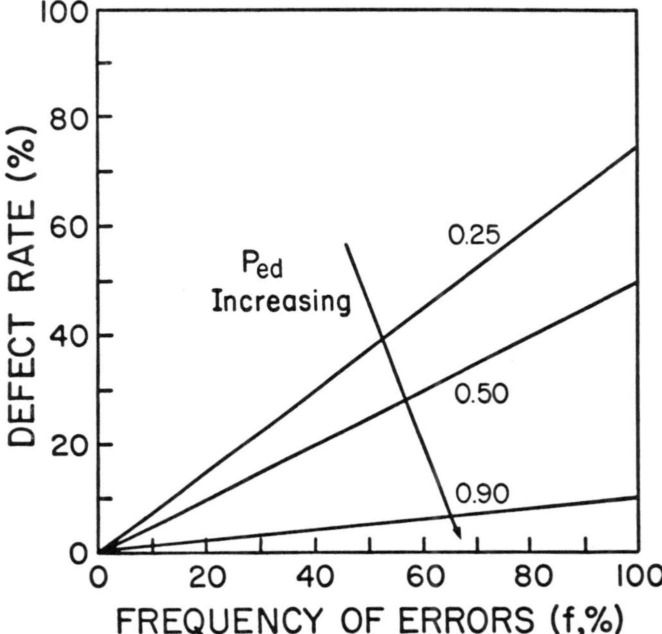

Fig. 5-3. Defect rate as a function of the frequency of errors in the measurement procedure

the defect rate, though it is easier to achieve a high P_{ed} when P_{fr} is allowed to increase.

Example application: urea nitrogen. Recall from Chapter 2 that the critical systematic error for the urea nitrogen example is 1.83s. In Chapters 3 and 4, the error-detection and false-rejection characteristics for the 1_{2s}, 1_{3s}, and $1_{3s}/2_{2s}/R_{4s}/4_{1s}/10_{\bar{x}}$ control procedures were described. The performance characteristics were compared in Table 4-4, which summarizes the information needed to calculate PV_r, PV_a, $PV_{r\&a}$, and the defect rate.

Table 5-3 shows the results of the calculations for the 1_{2s}, 1_{3s}, and $1_{3s}/2_{2s}/R_{4s}/4_{1s}/10_{\bar{x}}$ control procedures when applied to the measurement procedure for urea nitrogen. For each control procedure, calculations based on frequencies of errors of 0.00, 0.01, 0.02, 0.05, 0.10, 0.20, and 0.50 are presented. When f is 0.00 (i.e., when the measurement procedure is perfectly stable), the top row in each group indicates the correctness of the control signals and the quality expected for the analytical process. In this situation, a reject signal is always misleading, PV_r = 0.00, and an accept signal is always correct, PV_a = 1.00. The overall correctness of reject and accept decisions, $PV_{r\&a}$, is less

Table 5-3. Predictive Value Characteristics for Different Control Procedures with a Urea Nitrogen Measurement Procedure Having a Critical Systematic Error of 1.83s

Frequency of errors	PV_r	PV_a	$PV_{r\&a}$	Defect rate
A) 1_{2s}, N = 1, P_{fr} = 0.05, P_{ed} = 0.42				
0.00	0.00	1.00	0.95	0.00
0.01	0.08	0.99	0.94	0.01
0.02	0.15	0.99	0.94	0.01
0.05	0.31	0.97	0.92	0.03
0.10	0.48	0.94	0.90	0.06
0.20	0.68	0.87	0.84	0.12
0.50	0.89	0.62	0.69	0.29
B) 1_{2s}, N = 2, P_{fr} = 0.10, P_{ed} = 0.67				
0.00	0.00	1.00	0.90	0.00
0.01	0.06	1.00	0.90	0.00
0.02	0.12	0.99	0.90	0.01
0.05	0.26	0.98	0.89	0.02
0.10	0.43	0.96	0.88	0.03
0.20	0.63	0.92	0.85	0.07
0.50	0.87	0.73	0.79	0.17
C) 1_{2s}, N = 4, P_{fr} = 0.18, P_{ed} = 0.90				
0.00	0.00	1.00	0.82	0.00
0.01	0.05	1.00	0.82	0.00
0.02	0.09	1.00	0.82	0.00
0.05	0.21	0.99	0.82	0.01
0.10	0.36	0.99	0.83	0.01
0.20	0.56	0.97	0.84	0.02
0.50	0.83	0.89	0.86	0.05
D) 1_{3s}, N = 1, P_{fr} = 0.01, P_{ed} = 0.10				
0.00	0.00	1.00	0.99	0.00
0.01	0.09	0.99	0.98	0.01
0.02	0.17	0.98	0.97	0.02
0.05	0.34	0.95	0.95	0.05
0.10	0.53	0.91	0.90	0.09
0.20	0.71	0.81	0.81	0.18
0.50	0.91	0.52	0.55	0.45

(continued)

Table 5-3 (*continued*)

Frequency of errors	PV_r	PV_a	$PV_{r\&a}$	Defect rate
E) 1_{3s}, $N=2$, $P_{fr}=0.01$, $P_{ed}=0.17$				
0.00	0.00	1.00	0.99	0.00
0.01	0.15	0.99	0.98	0.01
0.02	0.26	0.98	0.97	0.02
0.05	0.47	0.96	0.95	0.04
0.10	0.65	0.91	0.91	0.08
0.20	0.81	0.83	0.83	0.17
0.50	0.94	0.54	0.58	0.10
F) 1_{3s}, $N=4$, $P_{fr}=0.01$, $P_{ed}=0.38$				
0.00	0.00	1.00	0.99	0.00
0.01	0.28	0.99	0.98	0.01
0.02	0.44	0.99	0.98	0.01
0.05	0.67	0.97	0.96	0.03
0.10	0.81	0.93	0.93	0.06
0.20	0.90	0.86	0.87	0.12
0.50	0.97	0.61	0.69	0.31
G) 1_{3s}, $N=8$, $P_{fr}=0.02$, $P_{ed}=0.57$				
0.00	0.00	1.00	0.98	0.00
0.01	0.22	1.00	0.98	0.00
0.02	0.37	0.99	0.97	0.01
0.05	0.60	0.98	0.96	0.02
0.10	0.76	0.95	0.94	0.04
0.20	0.88	0.90	0.90	0.09
0.50	0.97	0.70	0.78	0.22
H) $1_{3s}/2_{2s}/R_{4s}/4_{1s}/10_{\bar{x}}$, $N=2$, $P_{fr}=0.01$, $P_{ed}=0.33$				
0.00	0.00	1.00	0.99	0.00
0.01	0.25	0.99	0.98	0.01
0.02	0.40	0.99	0.98	0.01
0.05	0.63	0.97	0.96	0.03
0.10	0.79	0.93	0.92	0.07
0.20	0.89	0.86	0.86	0.13
0.50	0.97	0.60	0.66	0.34
I) $1_{3s}/2_{2s}/R_{4s}/4_{1s}/10_{\bar{x}}$, $N=4$, $P_{fr}=0.03$, $P_{ed}=0.74$				
0.00	0.00	1.00	0.97	0.00
0.01	0.20	1.00	0.97	0.00
0.02	0.33	0.99	0.97	0.01
0.05	0.56	0.99	0.96	0.01
0.10	0.73	0.97	0.95	0.03
0.20	0.86	0.94	0.92	0.05
0.50	0.96	0.79	0.86	0.13

than 1.00 by the proportion of false rejections that occur. The defect rate is always 0.00, regardless of what control procedure is used.

For a perfectly stable measurement procedure (f = 0.00), the choice of control procedure has no effect on the quality that will be achieved by the analytical process. Because no errors are occurring, the defect rate will be zero, even if no quality control is being performed. A cost-effective control procedure for this situation could be the 1_{3s} procedure with N = 1. Its error-detection rate is low, but large errors would be detected on the rare occasions when they occur. Its low false-rejection rate would minimize repeat work and therefore provide better productivity than the other control procedures.

As the frequency of errors increases, the correctness of accept signals becomes important in determining the quality achieved. PV_a depends almost entirely on P_{ed}. As P_{ed} increases, PV_a increases and the defect rate decreases. Different control procedures can achieve a given P_{ed} with different numbers of control measurements; that is, the same quality can be achieved with different Ns.

For example, if f = 0.10 (10%), defect rates of 3–4% can be achieved by using the 1_{2s} procedure with N = 2 (3%), the 1_{3s} control procedure with N = 8 (4%), or the $1_{3s}/2_{2s}/R_{4s}/4_{1s}/10_{\bar{x}}$ control procedure with N = 4 (3%). Although the quality of the analytical process will be nearly the same with these three control procedures, the productivity of the process would be expected to change according to the different PV_r values (0.43, 0.76, and 0.73, respectively) and the different numbers of control measurements required (N = 2, 8, and 4, respectively). Thus the 1_{2s} procedure would involve more repeat work, decreasing the productivity of the process. Use of a 1_{3s} or multi-rule procedure looks preferable, but the need for more control measurements with those procedures could offset the potential gain in productivity. The fewer control measurements for the multi-rule procedure make it a better choice because the productivity of the process would be expected to be better.

When the frequency of errors is very high, e.g., 20–50%, the only way to maintain a low defect rate is to use a control procedure with a very high error-detection rate. The 1_{2s} control procedure with N = 4 can keep the defect rate at 5% or less. Thus, despite its high false-rejection rate, the 1_{2s} control procedure may be the best choice for maintaining quality when f is high.

Estimation of Predictive Value Characteristics from Average Run Lengths

In the preceding section, the predictive value characteristics were estimated from the control procedure's probabilities for rejection, rather than average run lengths. As discussed in Chapter 3, the probabilities for rejection are the appropriate performance characteristics for assessing the detection of *intermittent* errors, i.e., errors that occur in an individual run but not necessarily in the subsequent runs. Average run length characteristics are the appropriate performance characteristics when assessing the detection of *persistent* errors, i.e., errors that, once they occur, are present in the following runs until detected and removed.

Table 5-4 summarizes the equations for calculating the predictive value terms from average run length characteristics. [See the addendum to this chapter for derivation of these equations.] The correctness of a control signal depends on the frequency of errors as described earlier. PV_r depends primarily on the average run length for acceptability quality (ARL_a), PV_a depends primarily on the average run length for rejectable quality (ARL_r). $PV_{r\&a}$ depends on ARL_a when f is low and on ARL_r when f is high.

The quality of an analytical process can be predicted by calculating the defect rate from the measurement procedure's frequency of errors (f) and from the control procedure's average run length for rejectable quality (ARL_r). The defect rate increases when the frequency of errors increases and when the average run length for rejectable quality increases.

Table 5-4. Predictive Value Characteristics as Functions of the Average Run Length for Rejectable Quality (ARL_r), Average Run Length for Acceptable Quality (ARL_a), and Frequency of Errors (f)

Analytical runs	Reject signal	Accept signal
With errors	$n_{tr} = n_t f$	$n_{fa} = n_t f\,(ARL_r - 1)$
Without errors	$n_{fr} = n_t\,(1 - ARL_r f)\left(\frac{1}{ARL_a}\right)$	$n_{ta} = n_t\,(1 - ARL_r f)\left(1 - \frac{1}{ARL_a}\right)$

$$PV_r = \frac{n_{tr}}{n_{tr} + n_{fr}} = \frac{f}{f + (1 - ARL_r f)\left(\frac{1}{ARL_a}\right)}$$

$$PV_a = \frac{n_{ta}}{n_{ta} + n_{fa}} = \frac{(1 - ARL_r f)\left(1 - \frac{1}{ARL_a}\right)}{(1 - ARL_r f)\left(1 - \frac{1}{ARL_a}\right) + f(ARL_r - 1)}$$

$$PV_{r\&a} = \frac{n_{tr} + n_{ta}}{n_t} = f + (1 - ARL_r f)\left(1 - \frac{1}{ARL_a}\right)$$

$$\text{Defect rate} = n_{fa}/n_t = f(ARL_r - 1)$$

Analogy to Predictive Value of Diagnostic Tests

For analysts who have been involved in evaluating diagnostic tests, the predictive value concepts presented here should seem familiar. The predictive value characteristics are analogous to certain characteristics that are evaluated when assessing the clinical usefulness of a diagnostic test (2). A "QC test" and a "diagnostic test" are similar in that both try to classify the subject being tested (an analytical run, in one case; a patient, in the other) into one of two classes. The quality-control test tries to classify analytical runs into those with and without problems (errors); the diagnostic test tries to classify patients into those with and without problems (diseases). The performance of both can be described in terms of true rejects (true positives), false rejects (false positives), false accepts (false negatives), and true accepts (true negatives).

The probability for error detection (P_{ed}) is analogous to diagnostic sensitivity. The probability for false rejection (P_{fr}) is related to diagnostic specificity, or more directly, is analogous to the false-positive rate, which is 1 minus diagnostic specificity. The frequency of errors (f) is analogous to the prevalence of disease. The predictive value of a reject signal (PV_r) is analogous to the predictive value of a positive diagnostic test, the predictive value of an accept signal (PV_a) to the predictive value of a negative test, the predictive value of both reject and accept signals ($PV_{r\&a}$) to diagnostic "efficiency," and the defect rate to the "false-negative rate" of a diagnostic test.

Although the similarities in the two predictive value models are striking, differences exist that must be understood. P_{ed} and P_{fr} are theoretical properties of the control procedure and can be estimated from probability calculations or computer simulation studies, whereas diagnostic sensitivity and specificity must be determined from carefully designed experimental studies. Estimation of f may be difficult because such data regarding an assay may not be readily available, whereas the prevalence of disease is often available in the medical literature.

The most important point of the analogy is that a control procedure can be optimized to fit the frequency of errors of the particular measurement procedure that is to be controlled, in the same manner that a diagnostic test can be optimized to fit the prevalence of disease in the particular patient population to be tested.

Implications for the Selection or Design of Control Procedures

The predictive value characteristics of an analytical process illustrate how the correctness of accept and reject signals depends on the frequency of errors occurring in the measurement procedure. When it is desirable to optimize the correctness of reject signals, then the probability for false rejection must be kept very low, or the average run length for acceptable quality must be long. When it is desirable to optimize the correctness of accept signals, then the probability for error detection must be high, or the average run length for rejectable quality must be short. When both are desired, an ideal control procedure is required, which will likely need a large number of control measurements and be a costly procedure.

Select "low-f" and "high-f" control procedures. Presumably, different designs of control procedures are appropriate for measurement procedures with different frequencies of error. For a measurement procedure having a low frequency of errors, it is advisable to optimize the interpretation of reject signals (a low-f design). Otherwise, false rejections will result in costly and ineffective control. For a measurement procedure having a high frequency of errors, one should optimize the interpretation of accept signals (a high-f design), to minimize the number of falsely accepted runs (i.e., to avoid reporting runs having errors).

A low-f design would have few false rejections and a low to moderate rate of error detection. A 1_{3s} control procedure would be appropriate when f is low. For N = 1 to 4, the 1_{3s} control procedure would provide few false rejections and low to moderate error detection. A 1_{2s} procedure would not be satisfactory because of the many false rejections.

A high-f design would have a high rate of error detection, with secondary concern for the number of false rejections. A 1_{2s} control procedure may be a practical way to achieve high error detection with a low number of control observations. In this situation, false rejections are not as serious a problem as false acceptances. When a measurement procedure has a history of frequent errors, it is better to reject than to accept runs.

In applying this strategy, qualitative estimates of f will suffice, at least initially. The predictive value characteristics do not show large changes when the frequency of errors changes by only a few percent. It should be sufficient to simply identify stable and unstable measurement procedures, or situations with the potential for a high or low frequency of errors. Quantitative estimates of f could be obtained from quality-control records, particularly with the development of computerized control programs having database capabilities.

When new measurement procedures are being introduced, it is best, at first, to assume a high value for f and use a control procedure having a high rate of error detection. A realistic estimate of f can be obtained by monitoring the process during routine operation. On the basis of that estimate of f, one can then select or design a new control procedure. The analyst's objective should be to reduce f by implementing preventive maintenance procedures, which in turn will mean redesigning the control procedure as appropriate for the new, lower frequency of errors. Ideally, therefore, the selection or design of control procedures is a dynamic rather than a static process. Whenever f changes, new designs should be considered.

Design multi-stage control procedures. One can also use several different control procedures with a single measurement procedure, to respond to different frequencies of errors at different times in the routine operation of an analytical process. For example, a measurement procedure that undergoes many changes from day to day could be subjected to a "start-up" design with a high rate of error detection, followed by a "monitoring" design having a low false-rejection rate (once the start-up test has been passed). Still later, a "retrospective" design could be used to review control data covering a longer period during which many control measurements had been accumulated.

Figure 5-4 illustrates the kinds of power curves that would be desired for these different stages of design. The power curve for the start-up stage shows good error detection with some increase in false rejection, perhaps achieved by using a 1_{2s} control rule and two to four control

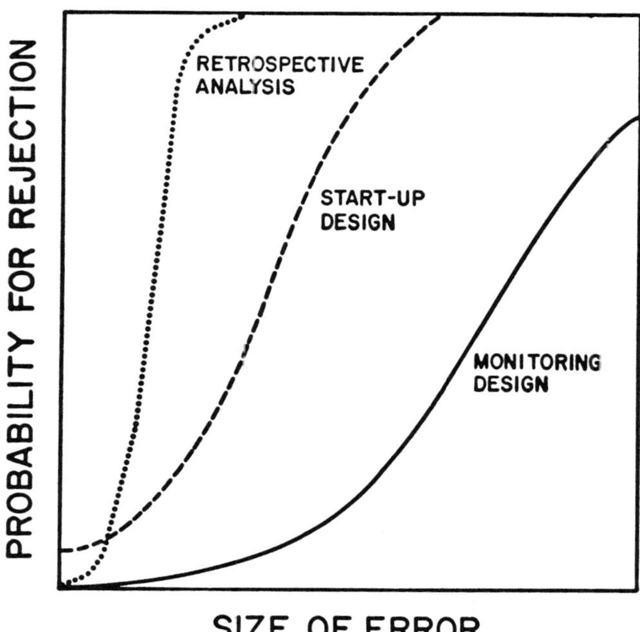

Fig. 5-4. Examples of power curves appropriate for different stages in a multi-stage control procedure

See text for details

measurements per run. The power curve for the monitoring stage shows very low false rejection and likewise low error detection; this performance could be achieved by using a 1_{3s} control rule and one or two control measurements per run. The retrospective design shows high error detection and low false rejection, and could be achieved by using multi-rule procedures having rules for consecutive runs, or by using mean and range (or chi-square) rules to test large numbers of control measurements.

Design an adaptable control algorithm. Using a general approach for implementing different designs of quality control can teach analysts a coordinated way to individualize the designs of control procedures. Several control procedures can be implemented, including multi-rule algorithms, mean and range charts (*3*), and trend-analysis techniques (*4,5*).

The multi-rule procedure discussed in Chapter 4 provides a general algorithm that can be tailored to different uses by choosing different rules and different numbers of control measurements. For example, for a start-up design, the use of N = 2 and the 1_{2s} rule as a rejection rule, instead of a warning rule, should maximize error detection. The 1_{3s} rule with N = 1 could be used for a monitoring design, minimizing false rejections. For retrospective analysis of control data, the 4_{1s} and $10_{\bar{x}}$ rules could be used.

Mean and range rules also provide a general way to individualize the designs by selecting the control limits to minimize the number of false rejections and selecting different numbers of control measurements to provide the desired error detection. At one extreme, a 1_{2s} or 1_{3s} rule could be considered a limiting application of a mean rule; at the other extreme, a large number of measurements could be incorporated into an estimate of the mean. Similarly, by using procedures for trend analysis (*4*), one can change the control limits and the number of control measurements to adapt the procedures for many different situations.

Summary

The quality of an analytical process and the correctness of the reject and accept decisions of a control procedure depend on the performance characteristics of the control procedure, as well as the frequency of errors, which is a characteristic of the measurement procedure. Because ideal control procedures having high error detection and low false rejection are costly, owing to their need for many control measurements, one approach to improving the cost-effectiveness of control procedures is to select or design the control procedure on the basis of the frequency of errors of the measurement procedure.

The quality expected from an analytical process can be predicted by calculating the defect rate from the error-detection characteristic of the control procedure and the frequency of errors of a measurement procedure. Similarly, the correctness of control signals can be predicted by calculating the predictive value characteristics as functions of the process characteristics (f, P_{ed} and P_{fr}, or ARL_r and ARL_a). The effects of different designs of quality control on the quality of the analytical process can be assessed to guide the selection or design of control procedures.

For *stable* measurement procedures, i.e., those having frequencies of errors of 1 or 2%, the control procedure should be selected or designed to have a low probability for false rejection (P_{fr}), or a long average run length for acceptable quality (ARL_a). Quality will be high, regardless of what control procedure is selected. Productivity is the main consideration in selecting the control procedure. A single-rule procedure such as a Levey–Jennings chart with 3s control limits and N = 1 will generally be adequate.

For *unstable* measurement procedures, i.e., those having frequencies of errors of 10% or greater, the control procedure should be selected or designed to have a high probability for error detection (P_{ed}) or a short average run length for rejectable quality (ARL_r). Quality will be high only if the control procedure has high capabilites for error detection. A single-rule procedure such as a Levey–Jennings chart with 2s control limits and with N = 2 to 4 should be sufficient. The greater false-rejection rate must be tolerated for the sake of high rates of error detection with use of only a few control measurements.

For measurement procedures having frequencies of errors from 2–3% to 5–10%, the control procedure should be selected or designed to maintain moderate error detection and reasonably low rates of false rejection. A multi-rule procedure with N = 2 to 4 should be adequate.

References

1. Westgard JO, Groth T. A predictive value model for quality control: effects of the prevalence of errors on the performance of control procedures. Am J Clin Pathol 1983;80:49–56.

2. Galen RS, Gambino RS. Beyond normality: the predictive value and efficiency of medical diagnoses. New York: John Wiley & Sons, 1975.

3. Hainline A. Quality assurance: theoretical and practical aspects. Selected Methods Clin Chem 1982;9:17–31.

4. Cembrowski GS, Westgard JO, Eggert AA, Toren EC Jr. Trend detection in control data: optimization and interpretation of Trigg's technique for trend analysis. Clin Chem 1975;21:1396–405.

5. Westgard JO, Groth T. Design and evaluation of statistical control procedures: applications of a computer "Quality Control Simulator" program. Clin Chem 1981;27:1536–45.

Addendum: Calculation of Predictive Value Characteristics

The predictive value characteristics of an analytical process can be calculated from the frequency of errors of a measurement procedure and the error-detection and false-rejection characteristics of a control procedure, either as probabilities for rejection or as average run lengths.

Calculation from Probabilities for Rejection

To express the numbers of runs in each class as functions of the performance characteristics of the analytical process, let n_e be the number of runs having errors and n_t be the total number of runs ($n_t = n_{tr} + n_{fr} + n_{fa} + n_{ta}$). Then the number of runs in each class is given by the following expressions:

$$n_{tr} = n_e P_{ed} \tag{5-1}$$

$$n_{fr} = (n_t - n_e) P_{fr} \tag{5-2}$$

$$n_{fa} = n_e - n_{tr} = n_e - n_e P_{ed} = n_e(1 - P_{ed}) \tag{5-3}$$

$$n_{ta} = (n_t - n_e)\ (1 - P_{fr}) \tag{5-4}$$

Furthermore, for an analytical process subject to intermittent errors, n_e and n_t can be expressed as a ratio, f, the frequency of occurrence of medically important errors:

$$f = n_e/n_t \tag{5-5}$$

Solving equation 5-5 for n_e gives:

$$n_e = n_t f \tag{5-6}$$

Substitution for n_e in equations 5-1 through 5-4 allows the number of runs in each class to be expressed as a function of the total number of runs (n_t) and of the characteristics of the analytical process (f, P_{ed}, P_{fr}).

$$n_{tr} = n_t f P_{ed} \tag{5-7}$$

$$n_{fr} = n_t(1 - f) P_{fr} \tag{5-8}$$

$$n_{fa} = n_t f(1 - P_{ed}) \tag{5-9}$$

$$n_{ta} = n_t(1 - f)(1 - P_{fr}) \tag{5-10}$$

By substituting these expressions for n_{tr}, n_{fr}, n_{fa}, and n_{ta} in the equations in Table 5-1, we can express PV_r, PV_a, $PV_{r\&a}$, and the defect rate as functions of the characteristics of the analytical process. For example, the defect rate can be expressed as a function of the process characteristics by substituting equation 5-9 for the number of false accept runs, as shown below:

$$\text{Defect rate} = n_{fa}/n_t = n_t f(1 - P_{ed})/n_t = f(1 - P_{ed}) \qquad (5\text{-}11)$$

See Table 5-2 for a summary of the equations for calculating the predictive value characteristics from the probabilities of error detection and false rejection of the control procedure.

Calculation from Average Run Lengths

To express the numbers of runs in each class as functions of the average run length characteristics, let n_e again be the number of runs with errors, which is a function of the total number of runs (n_t), the duration of an error (ARL_r, the average number of runs before an error is detected), and the frequency of the errors (f):

$$n_e = n_t ARL_r f \qquad (5\text{-}12)$$

Of the runs with errors, some will be true rejects and some will be false accepts. The number of true reject runs depends on f, because an error persists until it is detected:

$$n_{tr} = n_t f \qquad (5\text{-}13)$$

The number of false reject runs depends on the number of runs without errors ($n_t - n_e$) and the average run length for acceptable quality (ARL_a):

$$n_{fr} = (n_t - n_e)(1/ARL_a) \qquad (5\text{-}14)$$

Substituting equation 5-12 for n_e gives:

$$n_{fr} = (n_t - n_t ARL_r f)(1/ARL_a) = n_t(1 - ARL_r f)(1/ARL_a) \qquad (5\text{-}15)$$

The number of false accept runs equals the total number of runs with errors (n_e) minus the number of runs in which the errors were detected (n_{tr}):

$$n_{fa} = n_e - n_{tr} \qquad (5\text{-}16)$$

The number of false accept runs can be expressed as a function of process characteristics by substituting equations 5-12 and 5-13 into equation 5-16:

$$n_{fa} = n_t ARL_r f - n_t f = n_t f(ARL_r - 1) \tag{5-17}$$

The number of true accept runs equals the total number of runs minus those with errors and those falsely rejected:

$$n_{ta} = n_t - n_e - n_{fr} \tag{5-18}$$

Substituting equation 5-12 for n_e and equation 5-15 for n_{fr} gives:

$$\begin{aligned} n_{ta} &= n_t - n_t ARL_r f - n_t(1 - ARL_r f)(1/ARL_a) \\ &= n_t[(1 - ARL_r f) - (1 - ARL_r f)(1/ARL_a)] \\ &= n_t(1 - ARL_r f)[1 - (1/ARL_a)] \end{aligned} \tag{5-19}$$

Substituting these expressions for n_{tr}, n_{fr}, n_{fa}, and n_{ta} in Table 5-1 provides the equations for calculating the predictive value terms from the average run length characteristics of a control procedure. For example, the defect rate can be expressed as a function of process characteristics by substituting equation 5-17 for the number of false accept runs:

$$\text{Defect rate} = n_{fa}/n_t = n_t f(ARL_r - 1)/n_t = f(ARL_r - 1) \tag{5-20}$$

See Table 5-4 for a summary of the equations for calculating the predictive value characteristics from the average run length characteristics of the control procedure.

CHAPTER 6

Predicting the Productivity of an Analytical Process

To be cost-effective, a quality-control procedure should be selected or designed to maximize both the quality and productivity of an analytical process. In Chapter 5, we considered the effects of process characteristics on the correctness of control decisions and the resulting quality or defect rate, and developed equations to predict the defect rate of an analytical process from the characteristics of its measurement and control procedures. In this chapter, we discuss how the productivity of an analytical process depends on the characteristics of the measurement and control procedures.

We use the concept of "quality-costs," i.e., a broad view of costs that includes the costs of inadequate quality, to develop quantitative planning models that demonstrate how productivity depends on the measurement procedure's frequency of medically important errors and the error-detection and false-rejection characteristics of the control procedure. To predict productivity, we consider only those costs incurred at the process level, rather than extending the discussion to a more comprehensive assessment of laboratory costs or medical costs (which is beyond the scope of this book).

The type of analytical process becomes important in determining its productivity. Here, we will consider batch, simultaneous batch, and random access processes. In a "batch" process, a group of patients' samples are analyzed together with calibrators and controls in an analytical run. A "simultaneous batch" process has several batches being processed at the same time (in parallel). In a "random access" process, calibrators and controls are analyzed periodically and control status is established before the patients' samples are analyzed.

The Quality-Costs of an Analytical Process

The industrial concept of quality-costs, introduced in Chapter 1, is essential for understanding the cost components of quality, particularly the costs of not having adequate quality. Without this broad concept of cost, the only costs considered will probably be the costs of performing quality control, without including the savings produced by providing test results with the necessary quality.

Quality-Costs

The term *quality-costs* is generally used to describe the costs associated with producing a product with the quality necessary to satisfy the user or customer. As described in the industrial control literature (*1*), quality-costs are composed of prevention-costs, appraisal-costs, and failure-costs. "Prevention-costs" are incurred to prevent defects from occurring. "Appraisal-costs" are incurred to monitor the quality of the product. "Failure-costs" are incurred both internally, as "scrap" and "rework" costs, and externally, as costs due to "complaints" and "product services."

In clinical laboratories, the product is a test result. In applying the concept of quality-costs, we must consider the many quality-assurance activities that are required to produce a useful test result, categorizing the activities according to the quality-costs model. Elin (*2*) has reported the deliberations of a subcommittee of the College of American Pathologists, which defined the components of quality-costs in the context of a clinical laboratory and categorized many quality-assurance activities according to those definitions.

Prevention-costs are defined as those "expenses for developing, using, and improving a planned quality control program" (*2*). Activities include the assessment of medical needs, the derivation of analytical goals, and the general establishment of policies and procedures to meet those needs and goals, including the requisition of laboratory tests, collection of specimens, transport of specimens, verification of the status of the specimens before analysis, identification of specimens with potential interference problems, education and training of personnel, acquisition and maintenance of instrumentation, provision for the reporting and interpretation of test results, and many other related activities.

Appraisal-costs are those "expenses for the operation and maintenance of an internal (intralaboratory) quality assurance program and an external (interlaboratory) quality assurance program" (*2*). Activities include quality control of the analytical process, interlaboratory comparison studies, inspection and accreditation programs for the laboratory, monitoring of personnel and of instrument systems, and evaluation of reporting functions.

Internal failure-costs are those "expenses for reworking and/or discarding an entire batch of specimen results or an individual specimen due to some element of improper processing that leads to an erroneous result" (*2*). Included are costs for re-analyzing out-of-control runs, for troubleshooting analytical processes, and for assessing the frequency and sources of errors.

External failure-costs are those "expenses for the investigation of all inquiries by the physician or patient consumer as a result of the inability of the laboratory result to help solve the patient care problem" (*2*). These include the costs for investigation and correction of erroneous test results, as well as investigation of test results that cannot be properly utilized for any other reasons.

A general equation for quality-costs (Q-costs) is as follows:

$$\text{Q-costs} = \text{P-costs} + \text{A-costs} + \text{F-costs} \qquad (6\text{-}1)$$

where P-costs are prevention-costs, A-costs are appraisal-costs, and F-costs include both internal and external failure-costs. Prevention-costs and appraisal-costs are the costs most commonly included in the cost analysis of quality control, and are generally determined by calculations of direct and indirect costs. Failure-costs have rarely been included in the cost analysis of quality control because of the difficulty in determining them.

Failure-Costs

When selecting or designing quality-control procedures, it would be useful to be able to predict failure-costs from the characteristics of the analytical process. Such predictions can be made from a "model," which is simply a mathematical equation describing the behavior of the process as a function of its important characteristics.

Internal failure-costs are the costs incurred for those analytical runs that are rejected—both true reject and false reject runs. External failure-costs are the costs from false accept runs and sometimes from true accept runs, if physicians become suspicious of the quality of test results and re-order an assay to confirm previously reported results.

Failure-costs are the sum of the costs for the four classes:

$$\text{F-costs} = C_{tr}n_{tr} + C_{fr}n_{fr} + C_{fa}n_{fa} + C_{ta}n_{ta} \qquad (6\text{-}2)$$

where C_{tr}, C_{fr}, C_{fa}, and C_{ta} are the cost factors for the true reject, false reject, false accept, and true accept runs, respectively, and n_{tr}, n_{fr}, n_{fa}, and n_{ta} are the corresponding numbers of runs for each class.

Quality-Costs Models

We can obtain a general equation or model for quality-costs by substituting equation 6-2 into equation 6-1 (*3*):

$$\text{Q-costs} = \text{P-costs} + \text{A-costs} + C_{tr}n_{tr} + C_{fr}n_{fr} + C_{fa}n_{fa} + C_{ta}n_{ta} \qquad (6\text{-}3)$$

To predict the quality-costs of an analytical process, we can express the number of runs in each class as a function of process characteristics. Table 6-1 summarizes the expressions for all four classes. For *intermittent* errors, the number of runs is expressed in terms of the total number of analytical runs (n_t, equal to $n_{tr} + n_{fr} + n_{fa} + n_{ta}$), the frequency of errors of the measurement procedure (f), and the probability for error detection (P_{ed}) and for false rejection (P_{fr}) of the control procedure. For *persistent* errors, the number of runs in each class is expressed in terms of n_t, f, and the average run lengths for rejectable quality (ARL_r) and for acceptable quality (ARL_a) of the control procedure.

These expressions are the same as developed in Chapter 5, except that the expressions for the number of false-reject runs have been modified to consider simultaneous batch processes. Increasing the number of simultaneous batches increases the chance for false rejections for the process as a whole, just as increasing the number of control measurements increases the chance for false rejections. To express n_{fr} for a simultaneous batch process that is subject to intermittent errors, we replace P_{fr} in equation 5-8 with $1 - (1 - P_{fr})^m$, where m is the number of simultaneous batches or the number of channels in a multi-channel instrument. When m = 1, this term reduces to P_{fr} and the expression represents a single-channel batch process. When an analytical process is subject to persistent errors, we replace $1/ARL_a$ in equation 5-15 with the term $1 - [1 - (1/ARL_a)]^m$. When m = 1, this term reduces to $1/ARL_a$ and the expression represents a single-channel batch process.

Analytical processes subject to intermittent errors. Substituting the "intermittent error" expressions from Table 6-1 for the number of runs in

Table 6-1. Numbers of Runs in Each Class as Functions of Process Characteristics

	Expressions for calculation when errors are	
No. in class	Intermittent	Persistent
n_{tr}, true rejects	$n_t f P_{ed}$	$n_t f$
n_{fr}, false rejects	$n_t(1 - f)[1 - (1 - P_{fr})^m]$	$n_t(1 - ARL_r f)\left[1 - \left(1 - \frac{1}{ARL_a}\right)^m\right]$
n_{fr}, when m = 1:	$n_t(1 - f)P_{fr}$	$n_t(1 - ARL_r f)\left(\frac{1}{ARL_a}\right)$
n_{fa}, false accepts	$n_t f(1 - P_{ed})$	$n_t f(ARL_r - 1)$
n_{ta}, true accepts	$n_t(1 - f)(1 - P_{fr})$	$n_t(1 - ARL_r f)\left(1 - \frac{1}{ARL_a}\right)$

m = number of simultaneous batches, or number of channels in a multi-channel instrument.

each class in equation 6-3 gives the following model for the quality-costs of an analytical process subject to intermittent errors:

$$\text{Q-costs} = \text{P-costs} + \text{A-costs} + n_t\{C_{tr}fP_{ed} + C_{fr}(1-f)[1-(1-P_{fr})^m] + C_{fa}f(1-P_{ed}) + C_{ta}(1-f)(1-P_{fr})\} \quad (6\text{-}4)$$

where P-costs and A-costs can be estimated from laboratory expense and budget records, and the other terms can be estimated from the process characteristics and the cost factors for the various classes of runs.

Analytical processes subject to persistent errors. Substituting the "persistent error" expressions in Table 6-1 for the number of runs in each class in equation 6-3 gives the following model for an analytical process with errors that persist from one run to the next:

$$\text{Q-costs} = \text{P-costs} + \text{A-costs} + n_t\left\{C_{tr}f + C_{fr}(1-ARL_rf)\left[1-\left(1-\frac{1}{ARL_a}\right)^m\right] + C_{fa}f(ARL_r-1) + C_{ta}(1-ARL_rf)\left(1-\frac{1}{ARL_a}\right)\right\} \quad (6\text{-}5)$$

The model is similar to the previous model, except that the probabilities for error detection and false rejection have been replaced by average run length characteristics, which can be calculated from probability terms, as described in Chapters 3 and 4.

Development of Productivity Models

Specific models can be developed to predict the productivity of an analytical process by interpreting quality-costs in terms of the costs of repeat runs and repeat requests. The costs of repeat analyses are losses in process output: thus, quality-costs models can predict the effective utilization of process output. In this way, the quality-costs of an analytical process can be presented in terms of "test yield," which is a measure of productivity.

Test Yield Formulation of a Quality-Costs Model

The test yield of an analytical process is the portion of measurements that are correct and reportable as patients' results; it should ideally be 1 (or 100%). The test yield of an analytical process can be decreased by losses for measurements performed for calibration and control purposes, losses for analytical runs having errors and therefore needing to be repeated, losses for analytical runs without errors but being repeated because the control procedure has misclassified the run, losses for analytical runs with errors being reported as accurate (leading to repeat requests to verify the test results), and losses for analytical runs without errors but having repeat requests to verify the test results. All these losses are the quality-costs for the process:

$$\text{Q-costs} = L_{cc}n_t + L_{tr}n_{tr} + L_{fr}n_{fr} + L_{fa}n_{fa} + L_{ta}n_{ta} \quad (6\text{-}6)$$

where L_{cc}, L_{tr}, L_{fr}, L_{fa}, and L_{ta} are the loss factors for calibration and control, true reject runs, false reject runs, false accept runs, and true accept runs, respectively.

Subtracting these losses from the ideal output of the process can provide an estimate of the process yield. The average test yield of an analytical process should therefore be equal to 1 minus the average Q-costs per run:

$$\text{Test yield} = 1 - (\text{Q-costs}/n_t) \quad (6\text{-}7)$$

Substituting equation 6-6 for Q-costs in equation 6-7 gives the following expression:

$$\text{Test yield} = 1 - [(L_{cc}n_t + L_{tr}n_{tr} + L_{fr}n_{fr} + L_{fa}n_{fa} + L_{ta}n_{ta})/n_t] \quad (6\text{-}8)$$

The test yield of an analytical process can be predicted by expressing the numbers of runs in each class as functions of the process characteristics (using the expressions from Table 6-1) and by defining the loss (or cost) factors.

Loss factors. Appropriate loss factors for batch and random access processes are listed in Table 6-2 (*4*). The loss factor for calibration and control represents the reduction in output due to the number of calibration and control samples that must be analyzed. The loss factors for true and false rejects are the repeat factors for re-analysis of runs that are rejected. The loss factors for false accepts accounts for the repeat requests from physicians who recognize that erroneous results have been reported. The loss factor for true accepts accounts for repeat requests from physicians who have become suspicious of the quality of test results and want confirmation before they accept the test results. Because the true accept loss will be related to the quality achieved, this loss factor includes the defect rate, $f(1 - P_{ed})$ or $f(ARL_r - 1)$, as a proportionality term.

The values assigned for the rerun factors will depend on the management policies of individual laboratories, and may vary from laboratory to laboratory. Within a given laboratory, however, the assigned rerun factors are likely to apply to many or even all of the analytical processes.

Table 6-2. Loss Factors for Batch and Random Access Processes

Loss factor	Type of process: Batch	Random access
L_{cc}	$\frac{C+N}{T}$	same
L_{tr}	$R_{tr}\frac{S_p}{T}$	$R_{tr}\frac{N}{T}$
L_{fr}	$R_{fr}\frac{S_p}{T}$	$R_{fr}\frac{N}{T}$
L_{fa}	$R_{fa}\frac{S_p}{T}$	same
L_{ta} [a]	$R_{ta}f(1-P_{ed})\frac{S_p}{T}$	same
L_{ta} [b]	$R_{ta}f(ARL_r-1)\frac{S_p}{T}$	same

[a] For processes subject to intermittent errors.
[b] For processes subject to persistent errors.
C, N, and S_p are the average number of calibrators, controls, and patients' samples in an average analytical run of T total samples ($T = C + N + S_p$); R_{tr}, R_{fr}, R_{fa}, and R_{ta} are the rerun or repeat factors for true reject, false reject, false accept, and true accept runs, respectively.

The rerun factors for true and false rejections will usually be 1.0. Analysts commonly repeat all runs when the control procedure indicates the run is out of control. Because false rejections cannot be distinguished from true rejections, all rejection signals are managed alike.

The rerun factor for false acceptances is usually 2.0. That is, we assume that a physician re-orders the test, gets a repeat result that differs from the original result, and then re-orders again to determine which of the first two results is correct. The rerun factor for true acceptances would be 1.0 because the result of the reorder should agree with the original result.

Test yield models. Models for predicting the test yield of an analytical process as a function of process characteristics can be obtained by substituting the expressions from Table 6-1 and the loss or cost factors from Table 6-2 into equation 6-8. Models for batch and random access processes subject to intermittent or persistent analytical errors are described by the equations in Table 6-3. Again, C, N, and S_p are the average number of calibrators, controls, and patients' samples in an average analytical run having T total samples ($T = C + N + S_p$); R_{tr}, R_{fr}, R_{fa}, and R_{ta} are the appropriate rerun or repeat factors (see above); m is the number of simultaneous batches or channels in a multi-channel

Table 6-3. Productivity Models for Batch and Random Access Processes Subject to Intermittent and Persistent Errors

Batch process subject to intermittent errors

$$\text{Test yield} = 1 - \frac{C+N}{T} - \frac{S_p}{T}\Big\{R_{tr}fP_{ed} + R_{fr}(1-f)[1-(1-P_{fr})^m] + R_{fa}f(1-P_{ed}) + R_{ta}f(1-P_{ed})(1-f)(1-P_{fr})\Big\}$$

Random access process subject to intermittent errors

$$\text{Test yield} = 1 - \frac{C+N}{T} - \frac{N}{T}\Big[R_{tr}fP_{ed} + R_{fr}(1-f)P_{fr}\Big] - \frac{S_p}{T}\Big[R_{fa}f(1-P_{ed}) + R_{ta}f(1-P_{ed})(1-f)(1-P_{fr})\Big]$$

Batch process subject to persistent errors

$$\text{Test yield} = 1 - \frac{C+N}{T} - \frac{S_p}{T}\Big\{R_{tr}f + R_{fr}(1-ARL_rf)\Big[1-\Big(1-\frac{1}{ARL_a}\Big)^m\Big] + R_{fa}f(ARL_r-1) + R_{ta}f(ARL_r-1)(1-ARL_rf)\Big(1-\frac{1}{ARL_a}\Big)\Big\}$$

Random access process subject to persistent errors

$$\text{Test yield} = 1 - \frac{C+N}{T} - \frac{N}{T}\Big[R_{tr}f + R_{fr}(1-ARL_rf)\Big(\frac{1}{ARL_a}\Big)\Big] - \frac{S_p}{T}\Big[R_{fa}f(ARL_r-1) + R_{ta}f(ARL_r-1)(1-ARL_rf)\Big(1-\frac{1}{ARL_a}\Big)\Big]$$

process; f is the frequency of errors for the measurement procedure; and P_{ed}, P_{fr}, ARL_r, and ARL_a are as defined before.

Example Application: Factors Affecting Test Yield

To illustrate how the productivity of an analytical process depends on many factors, we have used these models to calculate test yield for many combinations of factors. These calculations are easily performed with electronic spreadsheets (see Appendix III).

Figure 6-1 shows a plot of process test utilization vs frequency of errors. Productivity, in terms of test yield, is what remains after subtracting the losses from measurements for calibration and control (CC-loss), true rejections (TR-loss), false rejections (FR-loss), false acceptances (FA-loss), and true acceptances (TA-loss).

Frequency of errors of the measurement procedure. The major factor affecting

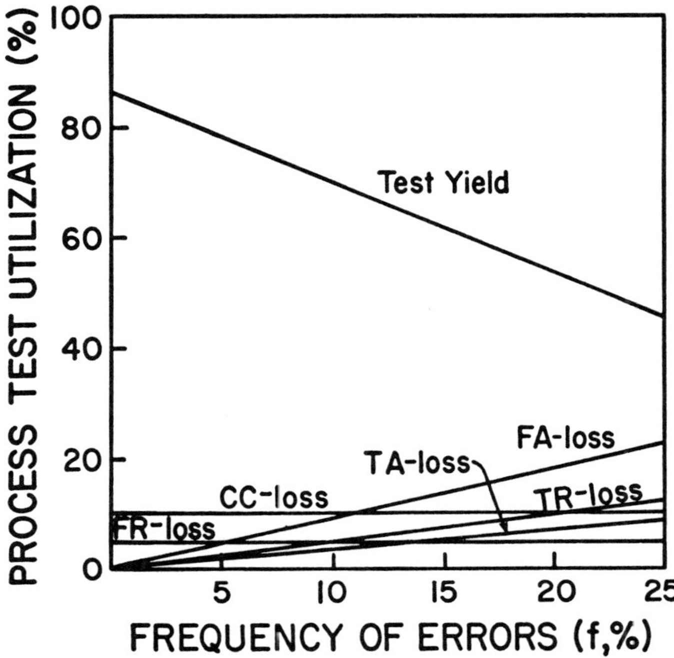

Fig. 6-1. The test utilization of a batch analytical process that is subject to intermittent analytical errors, as a function of the frequency of errors (f): C = 1, N = 1, $S_p = 28$, $P_{ed} = 0.50$, $P_{fr} = 0.05$, $R_{tr} = R_{fr} = 1.0$, $R_{fa} = 2.0$, $R_{ta} = 1.0$

Loss components shown are for calibration and control (CC-loss), true reject runs (TR-loss), false reject runs (FR-loss), false accept runs (FA-loss), and true accept runs (TA-loss). Test yield is the portion of measurements remaining after the losses are subtracted

the test yield of an analytical process is the frequency of errors of the measurement procedure. As Figure 6-1 shows, the highest test yield is obtained when the frequency of errors is zero. When errors are prevented, i.e., when f = 0, test yield will be highest because true-rejection losses and false-acceptance losses are reduced. Productivity will improve when quality is improved (i.e, when f is reduced), confirming Crosby's premise that quality is free (see Chapter 1).

False-rejection characteristic of the control procedure. Test yield also depends on the false-rejection characteristic of the control procedure (Figure 6-2*A*). As P_{fr} decreases, the test yield improves because false-rejection losses are reduced.

Error-detection characteristic of the control procedure. Test yield depends on the error-detection characteristic of the control procedure. Figure 6-2*B* shows how, as P_{ed} increases, the test yield improves because false-acceptance losses are decreased. True-rejection losses increase

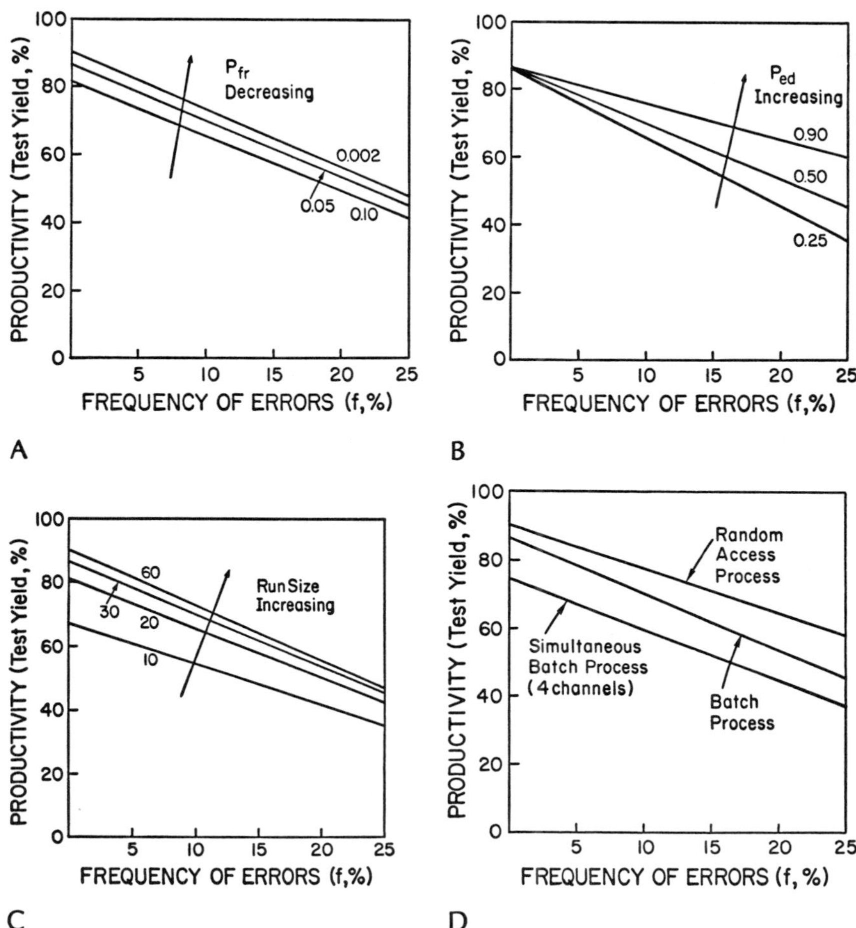

Fig. 6-2. Effect of (*A*) false-rejection rate and (*B*) error-detection rate of a control procedure, (*C*) run size, and (*D*) type of process on the productivity (test yield) of an analytical process

as P_{ed} increases but, because the rerun factor (or cost factor) for true rejections is lower than that for false acceptances, test yield will still improve.

Run size, and the number of calibrators and controls. The size of an analytical run would be expected to affect productivity because of losses for calibration and control samples. As shown in Figure 6-2*C*, increasing the number of samples in a run improves the test yield of the process, as long as the number of calibrators (C) and of control measurements (N) remains constant. Test yield also increases when C and N decrease, but the magnitude of such changes is small when the size of the analytical run is large.

Type of analytical process. Figure 6-2*D* shows the effect of different types of analytical processes, all for analytical runs of 30 samples (two controls, one calibrator, 27 patients' samples). With the same control procedure for all the processes (with $P_{ed} = 0.50$ and $P_{fr} = 0.05$), the test yield of a random access process would be higher than that of a batch process, which in turn is higher than that of a simultaneous batch process (four simultaneous batches or channels in this example).

Number of simultaneous batches. Figure 6-3 shows how seriously the test yield can be affected when the number of simultaneous batches (number of channels) increases. Our assumption in this model is that a run that is rejected will be repeated on the same instrument; the capacity of all channels will be consumed, even though only a single analyte may require a repeat run. Because the chance of rejecting a run increases as the number of channels or simultaneous batches increases, the false-rejection characteristic of the control procedure becomes a much more critical factor in simultaneous batch processes.

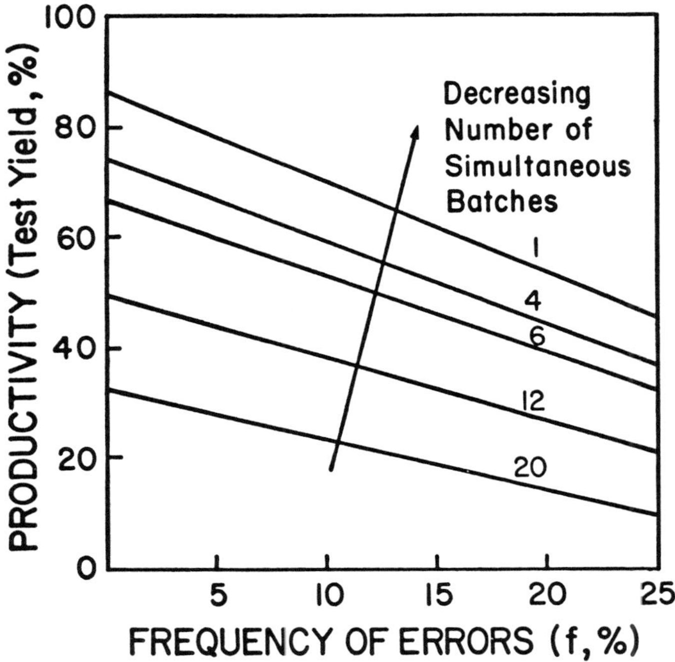

Fig. 6-3. Effect of the number of simultaneous batches on the productivity of an analytical process

Although a 5% false-rejection rate may be tolerable for a single-channel process, multi-channel processes require a much lower false-rejection rate. Alternatively, one can perform the repeat work with a different analytical process, so as to maintain the productivity of the multi-channel processor.

Quality–Productivity Planning Models

The calculations for defect rate from Chapter 5 are embodied in the model as false-acceptance losses, and can be provided along with the calculations for test yield to provide quality–productivity models for planning analytical processes. With these planning models, we can study the cost-effectiveness of quality-control procedures by predicting the defect rate as an indicator of effectiveness (related to quality) and the test yield as an indicator of cost (related to productivity).

Different control procedures can be expected to provide different defect rates and different test yields. When the frequency of errors is low, low defect rates or high quality is expected; high test yields or high productivity can be achieved by a control procedure that has few false rejections and a low number of control measurements. When the frequency of errors is high, high error detection is needed; in that case, analysts should select more-sensitive control rules or increase the number of control measurements. Changing control procedures or increasing the number of control measurements may actually improve both quality and productivity; therefore, careful selection or design of control procedures could result in improved quality at lower cost.

Example Application: Urea Nitrogen

Consider the measurement procedure for urea nitrogen with its critical systematic error of 1.83s, a requirement for an average of one calibrator per run (C = 1), and a run size of 30 (T = 30). Table 6-4 shows the effects of different control procedures on the test yield of a batch process, Table 6-5 the effects for a random access process. The expected quality of the process is given by the defect rate, as determined in Chapter 5 (see Table 5-3).

Assessment of the quality and productivity of analytical processes. Figure 6-4*A* presents the test yield and defect rate for the batch process controlled by a Levey–Jennings control chart with 2s control limits (1_{2s} control rule). The *y*-axis, "process test utilization," indicates the percent of process output that provides acceptable patients' results (test yield) and the percent of defective results (defect rate). The frequency of errors (*x*-axis) ranges from 0 to 25%. For a 1_{2s} control

Table 6-4. Effect of Different Control Procedures on Expected Productivity (Test Yield) for a Batch Process and a Urea Nitrogen Measurement Procedure with a Critical Systematic Error of 1.83s

Frequency of errors	CC-loss	TR-loss	FR-loss	FA-loss	TA-loss	Test yield
A) 1_{2s}, N = 1, $P_{fr} = 0.05$, $P_{ed} = 0.42$						
0.00	0.07	0.00	0.05	0.00	0.00	0.89
0.01	0.07	0.00	0.05	0.01	0.01	0.87
0.02	0.07	0.01	0.05	0.02	0.01	0.85
0.05	0.07	0.02	0.04	0.05	0.02	0.79
0.10	0.07	0.04	0.04	0.11	0.05	0.70
0.20	0.07	0.08	0.04	0.22	0.08	0.52
0.50	0.07	0.20	0.02	0.54	0.13	0.04
B) 1_{2s}, N = 2, $P_{fr} = 0.10$, $P_{ed} = 0.67$						
0.00	0.10	0.00	0.09	0.00	0.00	0.81
0.01	0.10	0.01	0.09	0.01	0.00	0.80
0.02	0.10	0.01	0.09	0.01	0.01	0.78
0.05	0.10	0.03	0.09	0.03	0.01	0.74
0.10	0.10	0.06	0.08	0.06	0.02	0.68
0.20	0.10	0.12	0.07	0.12	0.04	0.55
0.50	0.10	0.30	0.05	0.30	0.07	0.19
C) 1_{2s}, N = 4, $P_{fr} = 0.18$, $P_{ed} = 0.90$						
0.00	0.17	0.00	0.15	0.00	0.00	0.68
0.01	0.17	0.01	0.15	0.00	0.00	0.67
0.02	0.17	0.02	0.15	0.00	0.00	0.67
0.05	0.17	0.04	0.14	0.01	0.00	0.64
0.10	0.17	0.08	0.13	0.02	0.01	0.60
0.20	0.17	0.15	0.12	0.03	0.01	0.52
0.50	0.17	0.38	0.08	0.08	0.02	0.28
D) 1_{3s}, N = 1, $P_{fr} = 0.01$, $P_{ed} = 0.10$						
0.00	0.07	0.00	0.01	0.00	0.00	0.92
0.01	0.07	0.00	0.01	0.02	0.01	0.90
0.02	0.07	0.00	0.01	0.03	0.02	0.87
0.05	0.07	0.00	0.01	0.08	0.04	0.80
0.10	0.07	0.01	0.01	0.17	0.07	0.67
0.20	0.07	0.02	0.01	0.34	0.13	0.44
0.50	0.07	0.05	0.00	0.84	0.21	0.00[a]

(continued)

Table 6-4. *(continued)*

Frequency of errors	CC-loss	TR-loss	FR-loss	FA-loss	TA-loss	Test yield
E) 1_{3s}, $N=2$, $P_{fr}=0.01$, $P_{ed}=0.17$						
0.00	0.10	0.00	0.01	0.00	0.00	0.89
0.01	0.10	0.00	0.01	0.01	0.01	0.87
0.02	0.10	0.00	0.01	0.03	0.01	0.84
0.05	0.10	0.01	0.01	0.07	0.04	0.77
0.10	0.10	0.02	0.01	0.15	0.07	0.66
0.20	0.10	0.03	0.01	0.30	0.12	0.45
0.50	0.10	0.08	0.00	0.75	0.18	0.00[a]
F) 1_{3s}, $N=4$, $P_{fr}=0.01$, $P_{ed}=0.38$						
0.00	0.17	0.00	0.01	0.00	0.00	0.83
0.01	0.17	0.00	0.01	0.01	0.01	0.81
0.02	0.17	0.01	0.01	0.02	0.01	0.79
0.05	0.17	0.02	0.01	0.05	0.02	0.73
0.10	0.17	0.03	0.01	0.10	0.05	0.64
0.20	0.17	0.06	0.01	0.21	0.08	0.47
0.50	0.17	0.16	0.00	0.52	0.13	0.03
G) 1_{3s}, $N=8$, $P_{fr}=0.02$, $P_{ed}=0.57$						
0.00	0.30	0.00	0.01	0.00	0.00	0.69
0.01	0.30	0.00	0.01	0.01	0.00	0.67
0.02	0.30	0.01	0.01	0.01	0.01	0.66
0.05	0.30	0.02	0.01	0.03	0.01	0.62
0.10	0.30	0.04	0.01	0.06	0.03	0.56
0.20	0.30	0.08	0.01	0.12	0.05	0.44
0.50	0.30	0.20	0.01	0.30	0.07	0.12
H) $1_{3s}/2_{2s}/R_{4s}/4_{1s}/10_{\bar{x}}$, $N=2$, $P_{fr}=0.01$, $P_{ed}=0.33$						
0.00	0.10	0.00	0.01	0.00	0.00	0.89
0.01	0.10	0.00	0.01	0.01	0.01	0.87
0.02	0.10	0.01	0.01	0.02	0.01	0.85
0.05	0.10	0.01	0.01	0.06	0.03	0.79
0.10	0.10	0.03	0.01	0.12	0.05	0.69
0.20	0.10	0.06	0.01	0.24	0.10	0.50
0.50	0.10	0.15	0.00	0.60	0.15	0.00[a]
I) $1_{3s}/2_{2s}/R_{4s}/4_{1s}/10_{\bar{x}}$, $N=4$, $P_{fr}=0.03$, $P_{ed}=0.74$						
0.00	0.17	0.00	0.03	0.00	0.00	0.81
0.01	0.17	0.01	0.02	0.00	0.00	0.80
0.02	0.17	0.01	0.02	0.01	0.00	0.78
0.05	0.17	0.03	0.02	0.02	0.01	0.75
0.10	0.17	0.06	0.02	0.04	0.02	0.69
0.20	0.17	0.12	0.02	0.09	0.03	0.57
0.50	0.17	0.31	0.01	0.22	0.05	0.24

[a] Losses consume all of process output, reducing yield to zero.

Table 6-5. Effect of Different Control Procedures on Expected Productivity (Test Yield) for a Random Access Process and a Urea Nitrogen Measurement Procedure with a Critical Systematic Error of 1.83s

Frequency of errors	CC-loss	TR-loss	FR-loss	FA-loss	TA-loss	Test yield
A) 1_{2s}, N = 1, $P_{fr} = 0.05$, $P_{ed} = 0.42$						
0.00	0.07	0.00	0.00	0.00	0.00	0.93
0.01	0.07	0.00	0.00	0.01	0.01	0.92
0.02	0.07	0.00	0.00	0.02	0.01	0.90
0.05	0.07	0.00	0.00	0.05	0.02	0.85
0.10	0.07	0.00	0.00	0.11	0.05	0.78
0.20	0.07	0.00	0.00	0.22	0.08	0.63
0.50	0.07	0.01	0.01	0.54	0.13	0.26
B) 1_{2s}, N = 2, $P_{fr} = 0.10$, $P_{ed} = 0.67$						
0.00	0.10	0.00	0.01	0.00	0.00	0.89
0.01	0.10	0.00	0.01	0.01	0.00	0.88
0.02	0.10	0.00	0.01	0.01	0.01	0.88
0.05	0.10	0.00	0.01	0.03	0.01	0.85
0.10	0.10	0.01	0.01	0.06	0.02	0.81
0.20	0.10	0.01	0.01	0.12	0.04	0.72
0.50	0.10	0.02	0.01	0.30	0.07	0.51
C) 1_{2s}, N = 4, $P_{fr} = 0.18$, $P_{ed} = 0.90$						
0.00	0.17	0.00	0.02	0.00	0.00	0.81
0.01	0.17	0.00	0.02	0.00	0.00	0.81
0.02	0.17	0.00	0.02	0.00	0.00	0.80
0.05	0.17	0.01	0.02	0.01	0.00	0.79
0.10	0.17	0.01	0.02	0.02	0.01	0.78
0.20	0.17	0.02	0.02	0.03	0.01	0.75
0.50	0.17	0.06	0.02	0.08	0.02	0.66
D) 1_{3s}, N = 1, $P_{fr} = 0.01$, $P_{ed} = 0.10$						
0.00	0.07	0.00	0.00	0.00	0.00	0.93
0.01	0.07	0.00	0.00	0.02	0.01	0.91
0.02	0.07	0.00	0.00	0.03	0.02	0.88
0.05	0.07	0.00	0.00	0.08	0.04	0.81
0.10	0.07	0.00	0.00	0.17	0.07	0.69
0.20	0.07	0.00	0.00	0.34	0.13	0.46
0.50	0.07	0.00	0.00	0.84	0.21	0.00[a]

(continued)

Table 6-5. *(continued)*

Frequency of errors	CC-loss	TR-loss	FR-loss	FA-loss	TA-loss	Test yield
E) 1_{3s}, N = 2, P_{fr} = 0.01, P_{ed} = 0.17						
0.00	0.10	0.00	0.00	0.00	0.00	0.90
0.01	0.10	0.00	0.00	0.01	0.01	0.88
0.02	0.10	0.00	0.00	0.03	0.01	0.85
0.05	0.10	0.00	0.00	0.07	0.04	0.79
0.10	0.10	0.00	0.00	0.15	0.07	0.68
0.20	0.10	0.00	0.00	0.30	0.12	0.48
0.50	0.10	0.01	0.00	0.75	0.18	0.00[a]
F) 1_{3s}, N = 4, P_{fr} = 0.01, P_{ed} = 0.38						
0.00	0.17	0.00	0.00	0.00	0.00	0.83
0.01	0.17	0.00	0.00	0.01	0.01	0.82
0.02	0.17	0.00	0.00	0.02	0.01	0.80
0.05	0.17	0.00	0.00	0.05	0.02	0.75
0.10	0.17	0.01	0.00	0.10	0.05	0.68
0.20	0.17	0.01	0.00	0.21	0.08	0.53
0.50	0.17	0.03	0.00	0.52	0.13	0.16
G) 1_{3s}, N = 8, P_{fr} = 0.02, P_{ed} = 0.57						
0.00	0.30	0.00	0.01	0.00	0.00	0.69
0.01	0.30	0.00	0.01	0.01	0.00	0.68
0.02	0.30	0.00	0.01	0.01	0.01	0.67
0.05	0.30	0.01	0.01	0.03	0.01	0.64
0.10	0.30	0.02	0.00	0.06	0.03	0.59
0.20	0.30	0.03	0.00	0.12	0.05	0.50
0.50	0.30	0.08	0.00	0.30	0.07	0.25
H) $1_{3s}/2_{2s}/R_{4s}/4_{1s}/10_{\bar{x}}$, N = 2, P_{fr} = 0.01, P_{ed} = 0.33						
0.00	0.10	0.00	0.00	0.00	0.00	0.90
0.01	0.10	0.00	0.00	0.01	0.01	0.88
0.02	0.10	0.00	0.00	0.02	0.01	0.86
0.05	0.10	0.00	0.00	0.06	0.03	0.81
0.10	0.10	0.00	0.00	0.12	0.05	0.72
0.20	0.10	0.00	0.00	0.24	0.10	0.56
0.50	0.10	0.01	0.00	0.60	0.15	0.14
I) $1_{3s}/2_{2s}/R_{4s}/4_{1s}/10_{\bar{x}}$, N = 4, P_{fr} = 0.03, P_{ed} = 0.74						
0.00	0.17	0.00	0.00	0.00	0.00	0.83
0.01	0.17	0.00	0.00	0.00	0.00	0.82
0.02	0.17	0.00	0.00	0.01	0.00	0.81
0.05	0.17	0.00	0.00	0.02	0.01	0.79
0.10	0.17	0.01	0.00	0.04	0.02	0.76
0.20	0.17	0.02	0.00	0.09	0.03	0.69
0.50	0.17	0.05	0.00	0.22	0.05	0.51

[a] Losses consume all of process output, reducing yield to zero.

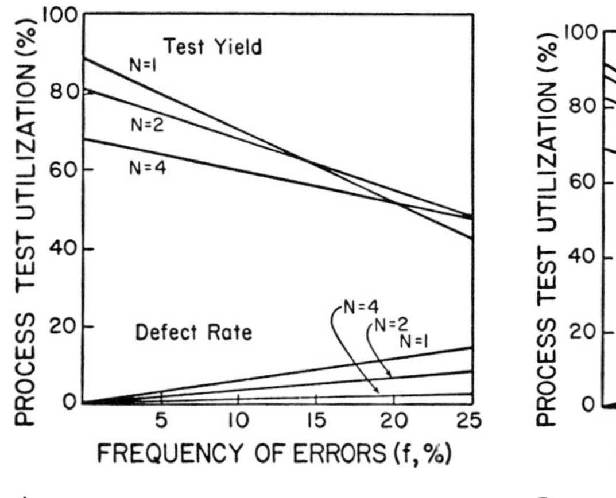

A

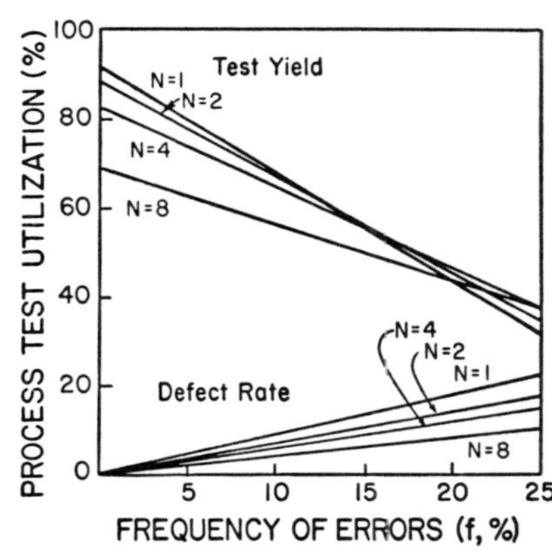

B

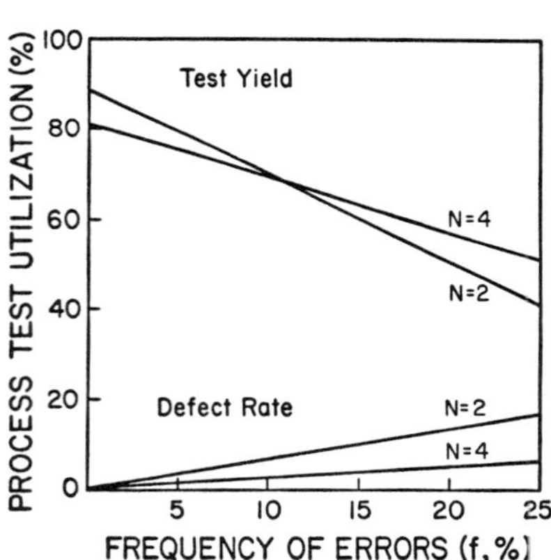

C

Fig. 6-4. Comparison of the test yields (measure of productivity) and the defect rates (measure of quality) for a batch analytical process and (*A*) a 1_{2s} control procedure with N = 1, 2, and 4; (*B*) a 1_{3s} control procedure with N = 1, 2, 4, and 8; and (*C*) a $1_{3s}/2_{2s}/R_{4s}/4_{1s}/10_{\bar{x}}$ multirule control procedure with N = 2 and 4

procedure, an increase in the number of control measurements (N) causes test yield to decrease when f is less than 15 to 20%. When f is greater, productivity increases as N increases. Quality also increases as N increases, as shown by the lower defect rates.

Figure 6-4*B* shows the behavior of the batch process controlled by a Levey–Jennings chart with 3s control limits (1_{3s} control rule). For f from 0 to 15%, an increase in N decreases the test yield; for f from 15 to 25%, the test yield does not vary much with N. Quality increases as N increases, but the defect rates are higher than observed for a 1_{2s} control procedure.

Figure 6-4*C* shows the behavior of a batch process controlled by a multi-rule control procedure ($1_{3s}/2_{2s}/R_{4s}/4_{1s}/10_{\bar{x}}$ control rules). When f is greater than about 10%, increasing N from 2 to 4 improves both the productivity and the quality of the analytical process.

The behavior of random access processes is given in Table 6-5, results for the 1_{2s}, the 1_{3s}, and the multi-rule control procedures being shown in Figure 6-5. The test yields achieved with a 1_{2s} control procedure in a random access process are considerably higher than those for the same control procedure in a batch process. For the 1_{3s} and multi-rule procedures, the differences in test yields between batch and random access processes are small when the frequency of errors is below 10%, but become more pronounced at higher frequencies.

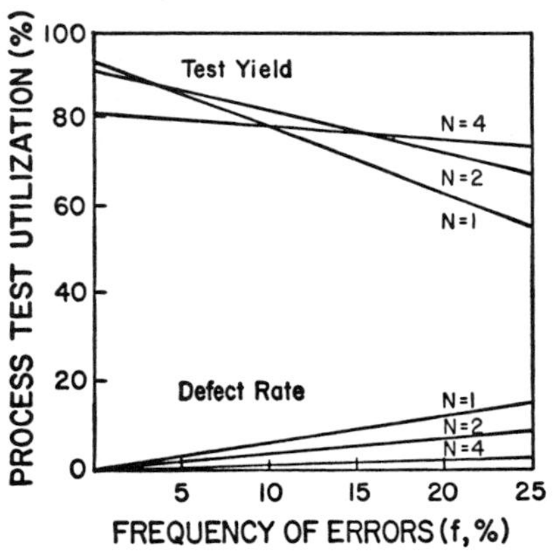

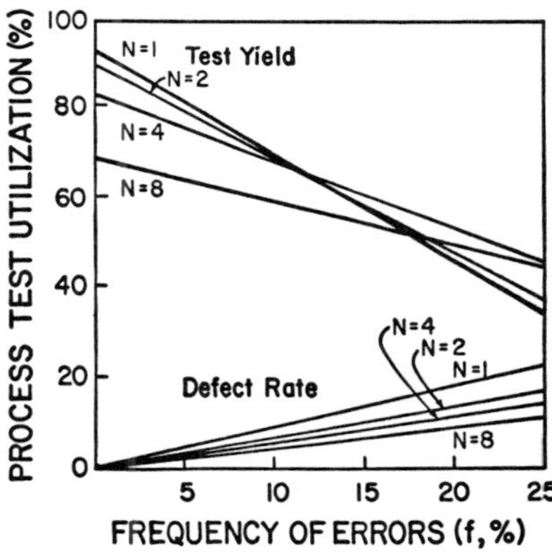

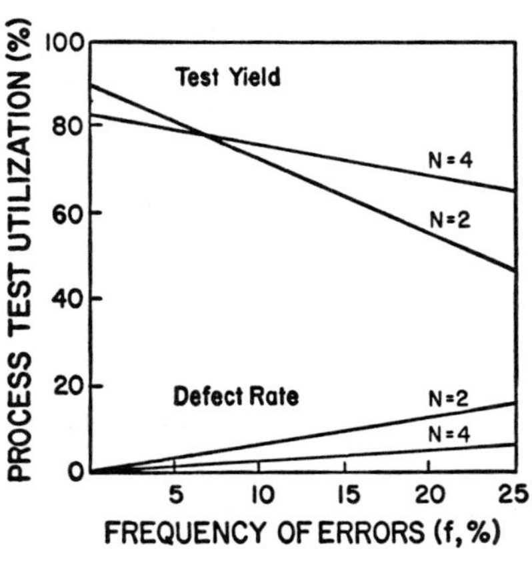

Fig. 6-5. Comparison of the test yields and the defect rates for a random access analytical process

A, B, C: control procedures and N values same as for the respective panels of Fig. 6-4

Comparison of cost-effectiveness of control procedures. The quality and productivity of the analytical processes controlled by the 1_{2s}, 1_{3s}, and multi-rule control procedures are compared in Figures 6-6 and 6-7. When N = 2 and f is about 12% or less, the multi-rule procedure provides the best productivity, but the quality of the 1_{2s} procedure is better; when f is above 12%, the 1_{2s} procedure provides the best productivity and the best quality.

When N = 4 and f is 2% or less, the 1_{3s} procedure provides the best productivity; quality will be very good for all three procedures. When N = 4 and f exceeds 2%, the multi-rule procedure provides the best productivity, but the 1_{2s} procedure provides somewhat better quality.

For a specified level of quality, say, a defect rate of 1% or less at f ≤ 5%, the multi-rule control procedure with N = 4 and the 1_{2s} control procedure with N = 2 provide the necessary quality and nearly the same productivities (Figure 6-7). A 1_{3s} control procedure, even with N = 8, does not provide as good quality and has a much lower productivity.

The cost-effectiveness of a quality-control procedure clearly depends on the frequency of errors of the measurement procedure. For a very stable measurement procedure (f = 0 to 1%), a 1_{3s} procedure or a multi-rule procedure with N = 2 is cost-effective. For error frequencies of 2 to 10%, the multi-rule procedure will provide the best productivity, but the 1_{2s} procedure will provide somewhat better quality. For f > 10%, the 1_{2s} control procedure with N = 2 and the multi-rule procedure

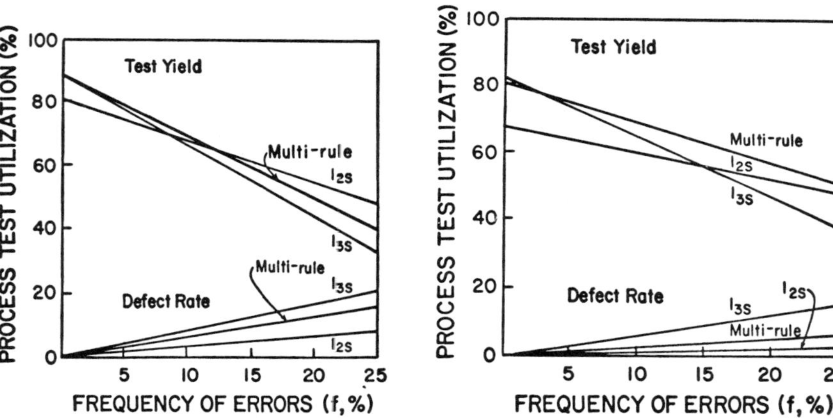

Fig. 6-6. Comparison of the test yields and the defect rates of three control procedures (1_{2s}, 1_{3s}, and $1_{3s}/2_{2s}/R_{4s}/4_{1s}/10_{\bar{x}}$ multi-rule) for a batch process subject to intermittent analytical errors

Left, N = 2; *right,* N = 4

with N = 4 provide comparable quality and productivity; for better quality, the 1_{2s} control procedure with N = 4 can be used.

Implications for the Selection or Design of Control Procedures

As illustrated in the discussions above, better quality and greater productivity can be achieved by the careful selection and design of control procedures. When the frequency of errors is low, it will be cost-effective to use single-rule control procedures with one or two control measurements per run. When the frequency of errors is high, control procedures with high rates of error detection are needed. Changing the control rules and increasing the number of control measurements can improve both quality and productivity.

Design for the type of process. The productivity of an analytical process depends on many factors, an important one being the type of analytical process—batch, simultaneous batch, or random access. The control procedure needs to be selected or designed for the particular type

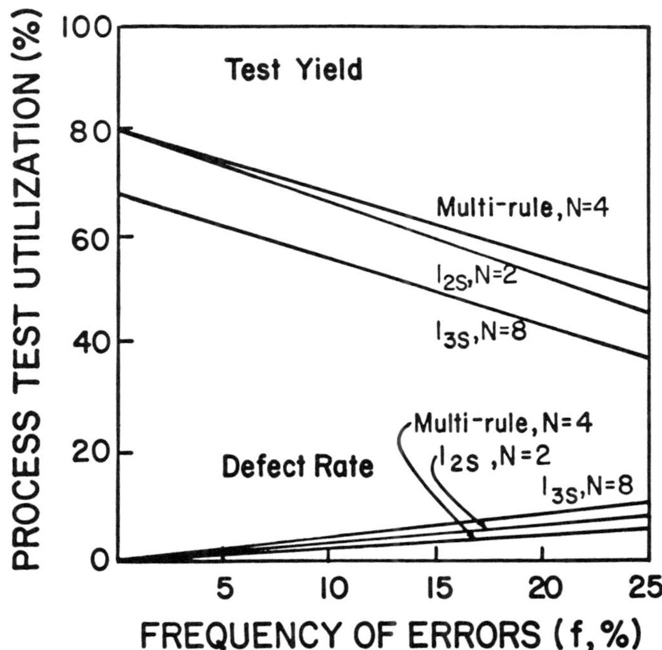

Fig. 6-7. Comparison of the test yields and the defect rates for the 1_{2s} control procedure with N = 2, the $1_{3s}/2_{2s}/R_{4s}/4_{1s}/10_{\bar{x}}$ multi-rule control procedure with N = 4, and the 1_{3s} control procedure with N = 8

of process. A lower probability for false rejection or a longer average run length for acceptable quality is required for a batch process than for a random access process. The productivity of a simultaneous batch process is especially affected, due to the increase of false rejections with an increase in the number of simultaneous batches (or with the number of channels on a multi-channel instrument).

Use quality–productivity planning models to study different designs. The effects of different control procedures on the quality and productivity of an analytical process can be studied by use of quality–productivity planning models. One must use a family of models to fit the characteristics of the many different analytical processes found in clinical laboratories. Models can be developed in the manner illustrated here. Use of "test yield" formulations provides more generally useful models than those involving more-comprehensive sets of cost factors. Implementation of the models on electronic spreadsheets with microcomputers can make the models easily available to laboratory personnel. The required information regarding the performance characteristics of control procedures can be obtained from computer simulation programs or from published power-function graphs, such as found in Appendix II.

Summary

The productivity of an analytical process can be described by its "test yield"—the portion of total analytical measurements that is correct and reportable as patients' results. Test yield depends on the type of analytical process (batch, simultaneous batch, or random access), run size to meet workload requirements, numbers of measurements required for calibration and control, the frequency of errors of the measurement procedure, the error-detection and false-rejection characteristics of the control procedure, and the laboratory policy on repeating runs that are out-of-control.

Productivity, in terms of test yield, can be predicted from quality-costs models when costs are defined as losses of measurements due to calibration, control, repeat runs, and repeat requests. The resulting quality–productivity models must take into account the type of analytical process and whether it is subject to intermittent or persistent errors. For intermittent errors, the model is best described in terms of the probabilities for error detection and false rejection. For persistent errors, the model is described in terms of the average run lengths for rejectable and acceptable quality.

In the technical management of analytical processes, quality–productivity models can be used as planning tools to evaluate the cost-effectiveness of different quality-control procedures. Through careful selection or design of control procedures, the laboratory may be able to achieve better quality at reduced costs. Cost-effective quality control requires that the design be individualized for the characteristics of the measurement procedure—particularly its frequency of errors, the nature of the errors (intermittent vs persistent), and the type of analytical process (batch vs simultaneous batch vs random access).

Without the careful selection or design of control procedures, the quality of laboratory testing may suffer under cost-cutting efforts. Laboratory managers and analysts must determine how their quality-control efforts can best be expended. More careful planning is required and can be aided by tools such as quality–productivity planning models.

References

1. Feigenbaum AV. Total quality control: engineering and management. New York: McGraw-Hill, 1961;83–9.

2. Elin RJ. Elements of cost management for quality assurance. Pathologist 1980;34:182–3, 194.

3. Westgard JO, Hyltoft Petersen P, Groth T. The quality-costs of an analytical process: I. Development of quality-costs models based on predictive value theory. Scand J Clin Lab Sci 1984;44(suppl 172):221–7.

4. Westgard JO, Hyltoft Petersen P, Groth T. The quality-costs of an analytical process: II. A test yield formulation of the predictive value quality-costs model. Scand J Clin Lab Sci 1984;44(suppl 172):228–36.

CHAPTER 7

Selecting and Designing Cost-Effective Quality-Control Procedures

Current practices of using the same control procedure for all measurement procedures in a laboratory cannot provide cost-effective quality control. Some measurement procedures will be over-controlled and some will be under-controlled. The right amount of quality control depends on each individual application, i.e., the analyte being measured, the medically required quality for that analyte, the characteristics of the measurement procedure (type, precision, accuracy, and stability), and the characteristics of the control procedure (error detection, false rejection). Cost-effective operation of an analytical process requires that a control procedure be selected or designed to fit the individual measurement procedure that is to be controlled.

In earlier chapters, we described the many factors that influence the cost-effectiveness of an analytical process and developed some ideas that should be useful for selecting or designing cost-effective quality-control procedures. In this chapter, we summarize those ideas and suggest some ways to apply them in your own laboratory.

Principles for Cost-Effective Quality Control

Principles presented in earlier chapters form the basis of our approach for selecting and designing cost-effective quality-control procedures. Here we review the most important ones to clarify our assumptions and beliefs.

Principle #1: The cost-effectiveness of a quality-control procedure is related to the quality and productivity achieved by an analytical process.

Approaches developed for quality management in industry clearly emphasize quality improvement as the means to improving productivity and reducing costs. Based on those approaches, "cost-effective" can be understood in terms of quality and productivity. "Cost" relates to productivity; "effectiveness" relates to quality. When applied to the use of control procedures in an analytical process in a clinical laboratory, a "cost-effective control procedure" is one that maximizes both the quality and productivity of an analytical process.

Principle #2: Quality should be understood as conformance to the requirements of the user or customer.

The users or customers for laboratory tests and services are primarily physicians, but also nurses, both acting on the behalf of patients, who are the ultimate consumers. By focusing on the user or customer, we can define the quality requirements for an analytical process and therefore have objective goals for evaluating the performance of the process. Quality has many dimensions, but it is concrete, definable, and measurable. The concern when selecting or designing cost-effective control procedures is the analytical quality that is necessary for medical use and interpretation of test results, i.e., the "medical usefulness" of the test results.

Principle #3: Quality requirements for analytical performance should be specified in terms of the medically allowable analytical error. A total error specification is preferable to separate specifications for precision and accuracy.

An analytical error is the difference or deviation of the test result from the true or correct value. Analytical quality is characterized by the size of the errors that occur. Although there may be random and systematic components of analytical error, it is the net effect or total analytical error that is important to the physician and patient.

Principle #4: Quality can be measured by the "defect rate" of an analytical process.

When analytical errors are large enough to be medically important (i.e., to affect the medical use and interpretation of the test results), the test results are defective and interfere with the diagnosis and treatment of patients. The number of defective test results, or the "defect rate," provides a measure of the quality of the analytical process. The defect rate is defined as the portion of patients' test results having medically important errors. The lower the defect rate, the higher the quality.

Principle #5: Cost should be understood in terms of "quality-costs," i.e., the total cost of quality, which includes the cost for prevention, appraisal, and failure.

A broad view of cost is essential; otherwise, the consequences of not having adequate quality control are overlooked. The industrial concept of "quality-costs" includes "failure-costs"—the costs incurred when a product or service does not satisfy the user or customer. Conventional views of cost tend to focus only on the cost of doing quality control, which is only the appraisal component of quality-costs.

Principle #6: Cost can be measured in units of productivity by the "test yield" of an analytical process.

The quality-costs of an analytical process can also be interpreted in terms of losses in process output, therefore permitting an assessment of how efficiently the process output is utilized. The "test yield" of an analytical process is the portion of measurements that are correct and reportable as patients' results. Test yield is derived from quality-costs, but presents the costs as a yield or measure of productivity.

Principle #7: An analytical process consists of a measurement procedure and a control procedure, and both have critical performance characteristics that can affect the quality and productivity of the process.

A measurement procedure is the part of the process that includes the protocol, materials, and equipment necessary for the analyst to obtain measurements of patients' samples. A control procedure is the part of the process that includes the protocol and materials that are necessary for the analyst to assess the validity of measurements on patients' samples to determine whether the test results can be reported.

The performance of a measurement procedure can be characterized by its precision and accuracy, and by the frequency and duration of medically important errors. High quality and high productivity are achieved when stable analytical performance causes only small, medically unimportant errors, and when occurrences of unstable performance are rare and brief.

The performance of a control procedure can be characterized by its capabilities for error detection and false rejection. High quality and high productivity are achieved when analytical runs are rejected only for the presence of medically important errors, and not for signals falsely generated by the control procedure.

Principle #8: An analytical process may be subject to random or systematic errors that may be intermittent or persistent in their duration.

Many possible error structures can be considered. We assume that errors are either random or systematic in nature. The sizes of the "medically important" errors can be determined from the total error specification and from the inherent imprecision and inaccuracy of the measurement procedure. The detection of these medically important errors will depend on their size and whether they occur only in a single run (intermittent error) or persist from run to run until detected and removed (persistent error).

Principle #9: The performance of a measurement procedure can be described in terms of its precision, accuracy, and frequency and duration of errors.

The stable performance of a measurement procedure is characterized by its precision and accuracy and is assessed from method evaluation studies. Precision is estimated from a replication experiment and described by the standard deviation. Accuracy is estimated from experiments to assess interference, recovery, and comparison of methods and is described by the average systematic difference or bias.

The unstable performance of a measurement procedure is characterized by its frequency of occurrence of analytical errors and the duration of those errors. Because these factors are seldom studied systematically, quantitative information about them is generally limited.

Principle #10: The performance of a control procedure can be described in terms of the probability for rejection for intermittent errors or the average run length for persistent errors.

The ability of a control procedure to detect a medically important error must be quantified, to guide the selection and design of control procedures. When the error is intermittent and occurs only in an individual run, the appropriate information is given by the probability for rejection of runs that have different sizes of errors. This information can be presented by power-function graphs: plots of the probability for rejection vs the size of analytical error occurring. Two power-function graphs are needed, one for random error and one for systematic error. When the error is persistent and lasts for several runs, the appropriate information is given by the average run length, which can be calculated from the probability information.

Principle #11: The quality and productivity of an analytical process can be predicted from the critical characteristics of the measurement and control procedures.

The defect rate and test yield of an analytical process can be estimated from the critical characteristics of the analytical process. Thus we can determine the effects of different control procedures on the expected quality and productivity of an analytical process.

To select the most cost-effective control procedure from a group of candidate procedures, assess and compare their defect rates and test yields, and select the procedure with the lowest defect rate (best quality) and highest test yield (best productivity).

To design a cost-effective control procedure, systematically study the defect rate and test yield by changing the control rules, the control limits, and the number of control measurements. The best design is the one that provides the lowest defect rate (best quality) and highest test yield (best productivity).

Guidelines for Developing Cost-Effective Control Procedures

The major concern in developing cost-effective quality control is to select or design a control procedure that is appropriate for the particular measurement procedure to be controlled. The general approach is to recognize the many factors that can affect the quality and productivity of an analytical process and include them when assessing the impact of different quality-control procedures.

Factors to be considered include the quality required medically, the stable performance of the measurement procedure (its precision and accuracy), the instability of the measurement procedure (the expected frequency of occurrence and duration of those errors), and the capabilities of a control procedure for detecting medically important errors.

The following guidelines outline how these many factors can be considered in developing cost-effective quality-control procedures.

Guideline #1: Define a total error specification based on the medical usefulness of the test results.

A rational starting point in the selection or design of a control procedure is the definition of quality requirements, with attention to the amount of analytical error that is allowable without invalidating the medical usefulness of the test results. A total error specification, or allowable total error, is appropriate for setting bounds or limits for the total amount of analytical error that can be permitted—bounds that include both the error due to the measurement procedure and the error resulting from the control procedure's lack of sensitivity.

The error specification should be customer oriented, representing the needs for medically useful test results. The physician survey approach recommended by Skendzel et al. (*1*) is an example of how the requirements for analytical quality can be determined from questionnaires. Other approaches and detailed examples are provided by Hørder (*2*).

As an example, for a urea-nitrogen measurement procedure, Ross

(*3*) recommends a medically allowable standard deviation of 16 mg/L, which we interpreted in Chapter 2 to mean a total error limit of 31.4 mg/L (1.96·16 mg/L).

Guideline #2: Evaluate the performance of the measurement procedure before selecting or designing the control procedure.

The performance of the measurement procedure is characterized by its precision and accuracy under stable operation, and its frequency of errors or occurrences of unstable operation. The precision and accuracy of the measurement procedure must be evaluated and found to satisfy the total error specification before you select or design the control procedure. The total error specification should be interpreted as a requirement for a 1% defect rate during stable operation (method evaluation) and for a maximum defect rate of 5% during unstable operation (calculation of the size of medically important errors). The quality specification needs to be interpreted more tightly during evaluation of the measurement procedure, to allow the control procedure a reasonable chance of detecting changes from stable to unstable operation.

A detailed example of the evaluation of a urea-nitrogen measurement procedure is provided in the monograph *Method Evaluation* (*4*). [Note that the total error specification was interpreted as a 95% limit or 5% defect rate in this earlier work, whereas we now recommend a 99% limit or 1% defect rate.]

Guideline #3: Calculate the medically important errors that must be detected by the control procedure.

The analytical errors that must be detected by the control procedure are those increases in a measurement procedure's imprecision or inaccuracy that could cause errors to exceed the total error specification. The sizes of the medically important errors should be calculated from the total error specification and the precision and accuracy of the measurement procedure (equations 2-3 and 2-7).

Medically important errors are defined here as those errors that would cause the maximum defect rate to exceed 5%. The critical random error (ΔRE_c) is the increase in standard deviation that would cause 2.5% of each tail of the error distribution to exceed the bounds set by the total error specification. The critical systematic error (ΔSE_c) is the systematic shift that would cause 5% of one tail of the distribution to exceed the bounds set by the total error specification. The control procedure should be selected or designed to provide the appropriate rate of error detection for errors of these critical sizes.

For a urea-nitrogen measurement procedure having a total error specification of 31.4 mg/L and a stable standard deviation of 9 mg/L, the critical random error (ΔRE_c) is a 1.78-fold increase in the stable standard deviation and the critical systematic error (ΔSE_c) is equivalent to 1.83s (see Chapter 2).

Guideline #4: Assess the performance characteristics of a control procedure by computer simulation when available, or, if unavailable, from documentation in the literature.

A computer simulation program (*5,6*) provides more general capabilities for assessing the performance characteristics of different control procedures by providing a greater variety of control rules and taking into account such factors as the between-run component of variation, data rounding, and the shape of the error distribution (*7*). When available, a simulation program provides a useful tool for assessing the performance characteristics and designing new control procedures (*8*). When not available, documentation in the literature should be sufficient for selecting control procedures.

Appendix II provides documentation for many of the control procedures commonly used in clinical laboratories.

Guideline #5: Select or design a control procedure to have high error detection and low false rejection.

Error detection depends on the decision criteria or control rules; it increases as the number of control measurements increase and as the size of the error increases. The size of error that is of most interest is the medically important error, an error large enough to cause the test result to be misused or misinterpreted. The ability to detect that error can be assessed quantitatively from power-function graphs, or from the average number of runs before rejection (average run length), which can be calculated from the probability information.

For a urea-nitrogen measurement procedure having a critical random error of 1.78 and a critical systematic error of 1.83s, power-function graphs for three commonly used control procedures were presented in Chapter 3. The probabilities for rejection and the average run lengths for the critical sizes of errors were determined in Chapters 3 and 4, and summarized in Table 4-4.

Guideline #6: Select or design the control procedure for the measurement procedure's expected frequency of medically important errors when a control procedure having both high error detection and low false rejection is impractical.

For small to moderate-size errors, control procedures having both high error detection *and* low false rejection are likely to require many control measurements per run (N), which is impractical in most service laboratories. However, one can select or design a control procedure to have *either* high error detection *or* low false rejection.

To provide a practical control procedure having a low N, select or design the control procedure for the expected frequency of errors, f. This characteristic describes the stability of the measurement procedure and its susceptibility to additional errors (i.e., errors in addition to the background random error or stable imprecision of the measurement procedure). Ideally, the frequency of errors would be zero, in which case the measurement procedure would be perfectly stable and there would be no need for a quality-control procedure. In practice, the frequency of errors is seldom zero and depends both on the measurement procedure selected and the preventive steps taken to assure that the procedure functions properly.

To optimize a control procedure for a measurement procedure having a low frequency of errors, select or design the control procedure to have a low probability for false rejection (or a long average run length for acceptable quality). A reject signal is most critical at low frequencies of error because it is wasteful to be repeating analytical runs when real problems are seldom occurring. The correctness of a reject signal depends primarily on the probability for false rejection (P_{fr}) or the average run length for acceptable quality (ARL_a). Correct reject signals are most easily achieved by maintaining a low P_{fr} or a long ARL_a. Increasing the error-detection capability of a control procedure is of secondary importance.

To optimize a control procedure for a measurement procedure having a high frequency of errors, select or design the control procedure to have a high probability for error detection (or a short average run length for rejectable quality). The correctness of an accept signal from a control procedure depends primarily on having a high probability for error detection (P_{ed}) or a short average run length for rejectable quality (ARL_r). There is little effect from P_{fr} or ARL_a.

For our urea-nitrogen example, the correctness of control decisions was assessed in Chapter 5 and presented in Table 5-3 for a critical systematic error of 1.83s. As shown, a simple 1_{3s} control procedure is adequate when the frequency of errors is very low (<2 or 3%); a simple 1_{2s} control procedure is advantageous when the frequency of errors is high (>10%). In between, a multi-rule procedure that can be implemented manually is useful.

Guideline #7: Use quality–productivity planning models to study more quantitatively how the quality and productivity of an analytical process will vary with the critical characteristics of the measurement procedure (frequency of errors) and the control procedure (error-detection and false-rejection characteristics).

In planning an analytical process and assessing the possible effects of different quality-control procedures on quality and productivity, we can use equations to predict the behavior of the analytical process as a function of critical characteristics of the measurement and control procedures. Quality–productivity planning models, such as those developed in Chapters 5 and 6, permit a more careful and more critical assessment of laboratory operation, particularly for selecting or designing quality-control procedures with consideration for the expected defect rate and test yield, and for the effects of the type of analytical process and the duration of analytical errors.

Consider quality in terms of defect rate. The number of defects depends primarily on how frequently the measurement procedure malfunctions and causes errors, and on the ability of the control procedure to detect those errors. Equation 5-11 shows how defect rate is related to a measurement procedure's frequency of errors and a control procedure's probability for error detection; equation 5-20 shows defect rate as a function of the control procedure's average run length for rejectable quality.

Consider the costs in terms of effective process utilization, or test yield. The cost factors depend on the extent or scope of which costs are to be included. Models can be developed to assess medical costs, laboratory costs, or process costs. The cost factors will also depend on the particular analyte, laboratory, and hospital application. A model can be expressed in chosen units of cost, absolute or relative, as appropriate for the consequences to be included. Costs in dollars may be appropriate for medical costs, whereas costs in work units may be useful for assessing laboratory costs. Other units are possible for more specific applications; for example, optimization of the analytical process itself may be based on the utilization of process output, i.e., costs in terms of the "test yield" of an analytical process (the portion of analytical measurements that are correct and reportable as patients' results).

Consider the type of analytical process (batch vs simultaneous batch vs random access). The cost or loss factors in quality-costs models depend on the type of analytical process being considered. For example, in batch processes, where control samples and patients' samples are analyzed together in a run, the repeat costs are high when a run is out of control because all patient samples have to be re-analyzed. In simultaneous batch processes, or multi-channel processes, rejections on one channel may impact on the operation of other channels, increasing repeat costs as the number of channels increases. In random access processes, control testing is performed before patients' samples are analyzed, thus minimizing repeat costs. Distinctions between types of processes will appear as different cost or re-run factors.

Consider the duration of the analytical errors. Intermittent errors occur in individual runs, but not necessarily in the subsequent runs. Persistent errors continue from one run to the next until detected and removed. Planning models must accommodate the different duration of the errors by describing the performance of a control procedure appropriately. For intermittent errors, the performance characteristics are described in terms of the probabilities for error detection and false rejection. For persistent errors, the performance characteristics are described in terms of the average run lengths for rejectable and acceptable qualities.

Implement planning models by using electronic spreadsheets. For performing the calculations required by the planning models, electronic spreadsheets provide a widely available and easy to use tool. Perform the calculations for a wide range of frequencies of errors, to obtain a general assessment of the expected quality and productivity as a function of frequency of errors.

Table 6-3 provided equations for estimating the test yield of batch and random access processes subject to intermittent or persistent errors. For our urea-nitrogen example, defect rates were given for several different control procedures and a wide range of frequency of errors in Table 5-3. Test yields were given in Table 6-4 for a batch process and in Table 6-5 for a random access process. Descriptions of spreadsheet programs for quality–productivity models are provided in Appendix III.

Strategies for Implementing Cost-Effective Quality Control

The principles and guidelines presented in the previous sections provide the background for understanding what cost-effective quality control means and how cost-effective quality-control procedures can be developed. There remains the question of how to put these ideas into operation in an individual laboratory. Finding efficient strategies will take effort (*9*). Some possible strategies are listed here, but this list is by no means complete and comprehensive.

Strategy #1: Select or design control procedures for individual analytical processes, not for general application to all processes in a laboratory.

We have repeatedly advocated the idea of "individualizing" the design of a control procedure for cost-effective quality control. That idea is the most important strategy. By selecting or designing a control procedure for an individual measurement procedure, we can incorporate the medical requirement for analytical performance, the measurement procedure's own imprecision (s) and inaccuracy (bias), the instability of the measurement procedure (f, frequency of errors), and the performance characteristics of different control procedures, but still keep the number of control measurements low and the control procedure simple enough to use manually. It is simply impossible to develop a universally applicable quality-control procedure that has perfect error detection, zero false rejections, only a few control measurements per run, simple statistical calculations, and manual charting.

Strategy #2: Target the analytical processes with the highest workload for the first applications.

The purpose is to apply the ideas to some processes where there could be some significant effects. Of the several hundred different tests and analytical processes potentially in use in a clinical laboratory, generally a relatively few account for a major portion of the workload; of those, most will have a history of few problems, but a few will have a history of many problems. These few high-workload processes with the many problems are the ones that first need their quality-control procedures optimized for quality and productivity. This strategy applies the "Pareto principle" of quality management: dealing with the few processes with the most problems will have the greatest impact.

Strategy #3: Start with qualitative rather than quantitative designs.

Begin by applying the general principles and guidelines qualitatively, based on your best judgment. The use of quantitative information—total error specifications, calculations of medically important errors, assessment of power functions, calculations of expected defect rates and test yields, etc.—may delay the application of the ideas. Start with qualitative applications, and progress to more quantitative applications.

Optimizing the quality and productivity of an analytical process is a dynamic rather than a static process; the control procedure will need to be changed as the preventive procedures reduce the frequency of errors. There is always an opportunity to further improve the design at a later time. What is important is to get started in applying the ideas.

Strategy #4: Provide in-service training in the principles of quality management to emphasize the prevention of problems as an essential activity for achieving cost-effective quality control.

The most cost-effective analytical process is one that never has any problems and therefore requires no quality control. Managers and analysts must understand the importance of permanently eliminating sources of problems, to increase both the quality and productivity of an analytical process.

Simple control procedures from qualitative designs are all that are needed when the measurement procedures are stable and few errors occur. Therefore, if the causes of errors can be removed or prevented, as mandated in industrial quality-management approaches, a qualitative design process and simple control procedures will be all that are needed.

Strategy #5: For stable instrument systems, particularly random access processes, analyze controls before analyzing patients' samples, instead of bracketing the patients' samples with the controls.

The repeat costs of false rejections are much reduced when controls are analyzed before the patients' samples, instead of along with the patients' samples. If the process is out of control, then only the controls themselves will need to be re-analyzed. Higher error detection can be achieved with fewer control measurements because more sensitive control rules with higher false-rejection rates can be used. This practice assumes, of course, that the process is very stable and does not change once its control status has been assessed. Many of the new instrument systems provide very good within-day stability and can be controlled differently from older systems—by analyzing control samples before patients' samples, instead of the older practice of "bracketing" patients' samples with controls. When the stability of the process permits, make instrument checks and analyze control samples to be sure the instrument systems are operating properly before analyzing patients' samples.

Strategy #6: Move any repeat work from multi-channel analyzers or simultaneous batch processes to a single-batch or random access analyzer.

The productivity of a simultaneous batch process cannot be maintained if the repeat work is performed on the same instrument system. There are too many false rejections, related to the effects of the simultaneous batches. If repeat work can be moved to a single-channel analyzer, then a control procedure can be selected or designed on the basis of single-channel performance. If repeat work is to be analyzed on the same multi-channel system, the false-rejection rate must be kept very low, often at the expense of reducing the error detection to an unsatisfactory rate.

Strategy #7: Adapt single-rule control procedures to different measurement procedures by letting the control limits change with increases in the number of control measurements and the number of simultaneous batches.

Single-rule procedures, such as Levey–Jennings charts with ±2s or ±3s control limits, have severe limitations—either too many false rejections or too little error detection. Control rules such as $1_{0.05}$ or $1_{0.01}$ allow the control limits to change as the number of control measurements per run increases, or as the number of simultaneous batches or channels increases. These control rules will have fewer false rejections than the 1_{2s} control rule and better error detection than the 1_{3s} control rule.

Strategy #8: Provide in-service training in statistical quality control so that analysts understand the technical details and performance characteristics of control procedures, and how the procedures are selected or designed for cost-effectiveness.

When control procedures are selected or designed for individual measurement procedures, analysts will become aware of different control procedures being used within a laboratory and will wonder why and how they have been chosen. Capitalize on these interests to establish a stronger background in statistical quality control, a better understanding of the performance characteristics of quality-control procedures, and an awareness of the many factors that are important in determining the quality and productivity of an analytical process. Objectives and guidelines from the literature (*10*) are suitable for quality-control workshops for in-service training courses for managers and analysts.

Strategy #9: Select or design an adaptable multi-rule control algorithm.

Whether working with qualitative or quantitative designs, different control procedures will be needed for different measurement procedures and types of processes, while maintaining a general approach that is understandable to all managers and analysts. A multi-rule algorithm can provide that general approach and yet be easily adapted to different applications. The general algorithm can provide moderate error detection *and* low false rejection. Appropriate adaptations can provide either very high error detection *or* very low false rejection by changing the control rules, the control limits, or the number of control measurements per run.

Strategy #10: When an analytical process is subject to persistent errors, select or design multi-rule control procedures that include control rules that utilize past control measurements.

When analytical errors are expected to persist from run to run, owing to the nature of the process or variables that affect the process, a multi-rule control procedure should include at least one control rule that utilizes data from previous runs. As the number of runs with error accumulates, the number of control measurements obtained under that error condition accumulates, increasing the error-detection capability of the control procedure.

Strategy #11: Select or design different control procedures for use during periods of stable and unstable operation.

There is no reason why only one control procedure should be available for use with a measurement procedure. When the measurement procedure is behaving in a stable manner, less control is necessary than when the measurement is unstable. During stable operation, use a control procedure having a very low false-rejection rate. During unstable operation (or when quality is suspect), use a control procedure having very high error detection, with little concern about its false-rejection rate.

Strategy #12: Develop multi-stage designs for routine use at different stages in the operation of an analytical process.

The stability of an analytical process may vary predictably, such that different designs of quality control are appropriate at different times or stages in the routine operation of the process. Such "multi-stage" designs may be sequential, switching from a start-up design to a monitoring design to a retrospective design, with a possible switch to an emergency or "stat" design when necessary. A multi-stage design may also have several control procedures operating in parallel to monitor segments of an analytical run for early identification of analytical problems, to evaluate runs for the purpose of data reporting, and to accumulate control information over several runs to identify smaller errors, initiate preventive maintenance procedures, and document the analytical quality achieved (*11*).

Strategy #13: Implement control procedures via computer when possible.

It will be easier to use individualized designs with different analytical processes and at different times in the operation of a process if the analyst is provided with the final "accept" or "reject" signal, without the need to remember all of the differences in the designs and make all the interpretations from the data. Although manual operation of individualized multi-rule, multi-stage control procedures is possible, this places demands on the analysts to remember all the details of the control procedure for each analytical process and each stage of application. At some point, computer support will become necessary for effective use of many "individualized" control procedures.

Computer-based quality-control programs should provide the flexibility needed by the manager and analyst to individualize designs for cost-effective operation of analytical processes. These programs should be capable of both on-line and manual data entry. Menus should permit selection of control rules, control limits, and the number of control measurements per run. Multi-rule procedures should be available, as should multi-stage designs. Interpretation features should be present, to help identify the type of analytical error encountered and offer suggestions for troubleshooting. Database capabilities for storage and documentation should be provided so that the frequency of errors can be estimated for the analytical processes. Summary analyses and reports should document the quality achieved by the process, assist in developing schedules for preventive maintenance procedures, and indicate when there are significant changes in the stability of the process and a need to redesign the control procedure. (A more detailed discussion of computer quality-control programs is given in references *12–16.*)

Strategy #14: Implement a broad program of quality management to place priority on quality improvement, productivity improvement, and cost reduction in all activities in the laboratory.

The principles and approaches incorporated in cost-effective quality control set the stage for broader application of quality improvement as a business strategy. Develop cost-effective quality control as part of the complete management strategy for the laboratory and the healthcare organization.

How to Get Started Doing Cost-Effective Quality Control

The selection or design of cost-effective quality-control procedures is an involved process because of the many factors that need to be considered. Understanding the principles and guidelines takes a lot of thought. Implementing the strategies takes a lot of planning. In short, it isn't easy. On the other hand, it isn't nearly as difficult as it may appear.

You can probably do something in your own laboratory right now to assess the cost-effectiveness of your control procedures and improve the operation of your analytical processes. Try the following to begin implementing cost-effective quality control.

- List the five analytical methods in your laboratory that have the fewest problems and the five methods with the most problems. Confer with analysts in the laboratory to see if your list reflects their experience, too.

• Determine what procedures are being used to control these 10 methods. If the same control procedure is being used with all of them, it most likely isn't cost-effective.

• Assess the error-detection and false-rejection characteristics of those control procedures. You can make a qualitative assessment on the basis of your knowledge of the performance of the different control procedures being used (control rules, number of control measurements), or you can make a more quantitative assessment by referring to the appropriate power functions in Appendix II. Assume that it would be important to detect a random error equivalent to a doubling of the standard deviation ($\Delta RE = 2.0$) or a systematic shift equivalent to twice the size of the standard deviation ($\Delta SE = 2.0s$).

It is very likely that you can improve cost-effectiveness by changing the control procedures used with your best methods to provide fewer false rejections and changing those used with your worst methods to provide better error detection. For your best methods, it may be as simple as reducing the number of control measurements, or changing to a Levey–Jennings chart with control limits set at $\pm 3s$ and using only one or two control measurements per run. For your worst methods, it may be as simple as increasing the number of control measurements, or changing to a Levey–Jennings chart with control limits set at $\pm 2s$ and having two to four control measurements per run.

Do it! Your applications of cost-effective quality control will grow once you get started.

Summary

The principles of cost-effective quality control reviewed above emphasize what cost-effectiveness means when applied to quality control in a service laboratory. A cost-effective quality-control procedure maximizes both the quality and productivity of an analytical process. Operational measures of quality and productivity are provided by an analytical process's defect rate and test yield, respectively.

The guidelines for developing cost-effective quality-control procedures outline a general approach for considering the many factors that affect the quality and productivity of an analytical process. The quantitative effects of many of these factors are illustrated by examples in earlier chapters. Quantitative planning models can be used to predict how the defect rate and test yield of an analytical process will be affected by different quality-control procedures.

The strategies for implementing cost-effective control procedures provide some practical advice on how to introduce cost-effective control procedures in a service laboratory. Some strategies that are relatively simple to implement may have large effects if applied to analytical processes that produce a major portion of the laboratory output.

With an understanding of the principles, guidelines, and strategies, you can make good judgments about the cost-effectiveness of quality-control procedures in your own laboratory and begin improving the quality and productivity of the analytical processes there.

References

1. Skendzel LP, Barnett RN, Platt R Medically useful criteria for analytical performance of laboratory tests. Am J Clin Pathol 1984;83:200–5.

2. Hørder M, ed. Assessing quality requirements in clinical chemistry. Scand J Clin Lab Invest 1980;40(suppl 155).

3. Ross JW. Precision performance standards: medical care and peer review criteria. Pathologist 1981;35:193–8.

4. Westgard JO, de Vos DJ, Hunt MR, Quam EF, Carey RN, Garber CC. Method evaluation. Houston, TX: Am Soc for Med Technol, 1978.

5. Groth T, Falk H, Westgard JO. An interactive computer simulation program for the design of statistical control procedures in clinical chemistry. Comput Programs Biomed 1981;13:73–86.

6. Groth T, Falk H, Westgard JO. A quality control simulator for design and evaluation of internal quality control procedures. Scand J Clin Lab Invest 1984;44(suppl 172):195–201.

7. Westgard JO, Falk H, Groth T. Influence of a between-run component of variation, choice of control limits, and shape of error distribution on the performance characteristics of rules for internal quality control. Clin Chem 1979;25:394–400.

8. Westgard JO, Groth T. Design and evaluation of statistical control procedures: applications of a computer "Quality Control Simulator" program. Clin Chem 1981;27:1536–45.

9. de Verdier C-H, Aronsson T, Nyberg A, eds. Quality control in clinical chemistry—efforts to find an efficient strategy. Scand J Clin Lab Invest 1984;44(suppl 172).

10. Westgard JO, Barry PL, Groth T. Workshops for teaching quality control to laboratory personnel: objectives and guidelines. Ibid.:215–8.

11. Westgard JO, Groth T, de Verdier C-H. Principles for developing improved quality control procedures. Ibid.:19–41.

12. Westgard JO, Groth T. Computer systems for implementation of internal quality control procedures. Ibid.:203–7.

13. Westgard JO. Better quality control through microcomputers. Diag Med 1982;5:60–74.

14. Westgard JO, Barry PL, Kurtycz DFI. Software considerations in the selection of a microcomputer quality control program. J Clin Lab Autom 1984;4:129–38.

15. Stewart CE, Oxford BS. Quality assurance programs and quality control data management. J Med Technol 1985;2:621–8.

16. Oxford BS. Statistical methods in quality assurance software. Ibid.:629–33.

Glossary of Terms

Definitions of important terms are obtained from documents of professional societies and organizations such as the International Federation of Clinical Chemistry (IFCC), the American Society for Quality Control (ASQC), and the National Committee for Clinical Laboratory Standards (NCCLS), or, in some cases, are based on our own use of these terms in the context of cost-effective quality control.

Accuracy. "Agreement between the best estimate of a quantity and its true value. It has no numerical value. See inaccuracy" (IFCC).

Analyte. The substance to be measured.

Analytical error. "Difference between the estimated value of a quantity and its true value. This difference (positive or negative) may be expressed either in the units in which the quantity is measured, or as a percentage of the true value" (IFCC). Used here to mean the difference between a patient's test result produced by the analytical process and the true value for that sample.

Analytical method. "Set of written instructions which describe the procedures, materials, and equipment, which are necessary for the analyst to obtain a result" (IFCC). Note that we use the term "measurement procedure," instead of "analytical method," to indicate clearly that the set of instructions applies to the measurement part of the procedure, rather than to the control part of the procedure.

Analytical process. The protocols, materials, and equipment required to produce a reportable analytical result. An analytical process has two major parts, a measurement procedure and a control procedure. The term "analytical method" is often used in a similar way, but that term is really a synonym for "measurement procedure" because the control procedure is not generally considered to be part of the analytical method.

Analytical run. As used here, that group of samples for which a decision is to be made concerning the validity of the measurements. The number of control measurements in that group is critical for assessing the performance characteristics of the control procedure. See also the following definitions by the IFCC and NCCLS.

IFCC: "This usually refers to a set of consecutive assays performed without interruption. The results are usually calculated from the same set of calibration standard readings. However, this definition may not be universally applicable, and in those cases the word series should be used after defining it."

NCCLS: "For purposes of quality control, an analytical run is an interval, that is, a period of time or series of measurements, within which the accuracy and precision of the measuring system is expected to be stable; between analytical runs events may occur causing the measurement process to be susceptible to variations which are important to detect. The length of an analytical run must be defined appropriately for the specific analytical system and specific laboratory application. The manufacturer should recommend run length for the analytical system (MRRL) and the user should define run length for the specific application (UDRL)."

Appraisal-costs, A-costs. That portion of quality-costs that is incurred to monitor the quality of a product.

Assignable cause. "A factor which contributes to variation and which is feasible to detect and identify" (ASQC).

Average run length, ARL. A performance characteristic of a control procedure that describes the average number of analytical runs that will occur before a run is rejected. Can be used for the situation where the only error present is the inherent imprecision of the measurement procedure (average run length for acceptable quality, ARL_a) or the situation where errors are present in addition to the inherent imprecision of the measurement procedure (average run length for rejectable quality, ARL_r).

"The average number of times that a process will have been sampled and evaluated before a shift in process level is signaled. A long ARL is desirable for a process located at its specified level (so as to minimize calling for unneeded investigation or corrective action) and a short ARL is desirable for a process shifted to some undesirable level (so that corrective action will be called for promptly). ARL curves are used to describe the relative quickness in detecting level shifts of various control chart systems" (ASQC).

Average run length for acceptable quality, ARL_a. The average number of analytical runs that occur before a run is rejected when the only error present is the inherent imprecision of the measurement procedure.

Average run length for rejectable quality, ARL_r. The average number of analytical runs that occur before a run is rejected when errors are present in addition to the inherent imprecision of the measurement procedure.

Batch analytical process. A type of analytical process where calibrators, controls, and patients' samples are analyzed together in a run. When a run is rejected and repeated, all patients' samples have to be repeated.

Between-run standard deviation, between-run component of variation, s_b. The standard deviation calculated from the averages (of several replicate measurements) from a series of several analytical runs. It describes changes that occur from one run to another, in contrast to changes occurring within a run, which are described by the within-run standard deviation, s_w.

Bias. Same as inaccuracy when referring to how a measured value compares with the true value. It also has a specific meaning in the statistical *t*-test or *Z*-test, where bias equals the difference between the two mean values being compared. Bias is generally used here as a measure of systematic error.

Calibration. "Process of relating the reading to the quantity required to be measured" (IFCC).

Chance causes, random causes. "Factors, generally numerous and individually of relatively small importance, which contribute to variation, but which are not feasible to detect or identify" (ASQC).

Chemical sensitivity. "The ability of an analytical method to detect small quantities of the measured component. It has no numerical value" (IFCC). This phrase is currently being replaced by "detection limit."

Chemical specificity. "The ability of an analytical method to determine solely the component(s) it purports to measure. It has no numerical value. It is assessed on the evidence available on the components which contribute to the result, and on the extent to which they do" (IFCC).

Clinical sensitivity, diagnostic sensitivity. A measure of how frequently a test is positive when a particular disease is present. Generally expressed as the percentage of individuals with a given disease who have a positive test result. Ideally, a test should have a sensitivity of 100%; i.e., the test should always give a positive result when the patient has the particular disease.

Clinical specificity, diagnostic specificity. A measure of how frequently a test is negative in the absence of a particular disease. Generally expressed as the percentage of individuals without a given disease who have a negative test result. Ideally, a test should have a specificity of 100%; i.e., the test should always give a negative result when the patient does not have the disease.

Coefficient of variation, CV. The relative standard deviation, i.e., the standard deviation expressed as a percentage of the mean [$CV = 100(s/\bar{x})$].

Confidence interval, confidence range. The interval or range of values that will contain the population parameter with a specified probability.

Constant systematic error. An error that is always the same direction and magnitude, even when the concentration of the analyte changes.

Control chart. "A graphical method for evaluating whether a process is or is not in a 'state of statistical control.' The determinations are made through comparison of the values of some statistical measure(s) for an ordered series of samples, or subgroups, with control limits" (ASQC).

Control limits. "Limits on a control chart which are used as criteria for signaling the need for action, or for judging whether a set of data does or does not indicate a 'state of control' " (ASQC). Used here to refer to the defined limits or ranges of results expected due to the random error of the method, and beyond which some course of action should be taken. It is common in clinical laboratories to use Levey–Jennings control charts with limits set as either the mean plus or minus two standard deviations, or the mean plus or minus three standard deviations.

Control material, control product. A control solution that is available, often commercially, liquid or lyophilized, and packaged in aliquots that can be prepared and used individually.

Control measurements, control observations. The analytical results obtained for control solutions (that are analyzed for purposes of quality control).

Control procedure, quality-control procedure. The protocol and materials that are necessary for an analyst to assess the validity of a measurement of a patient's sample and to determine whether a test result can be reported—that part of an analytical process that is concerned with testing the quality of the analytical results, in contrast to the measurement procedure, which gives the result. A control procedure is defined by its number of control measurements and its decision criteria (control rules) for judging the acceptability of the analytical results.

Control rule. A decision criterion for interpreting control data and making a judgment on the control status of an analytical run. Symbolized by A_L, where A is the abbreviation for a particular statistic or states the number of control measurements, and L is the control limit. An analytical run is rejected when the control measurements fulfill the stated conditions, i.e., when a certain statistic or number of control measurements exceeds the specified control limits.

Control solution, control specimen. "Specimen or solution which is analyzed solely for quality control purposes, not for calibration" (IFCC).

Cost-effective quality control. The use of a control procedure that maximizes both the quality and productivity of an analytical process. "Cost" is interpreted to mean productivity and "effective" is interpreted to mean quality.

Critical random error, ΔRE_c. The size of random error that causes a 5% maximum defect rate for the analytical process. Calculated as $(TE_a - \text{bias})/1.96s$, where TE_a is the total error specification, and bias is the inaccuracy and s the imprecision (standard deviation) of the measurement procedure.

Critical systematic error, ΔSE_c. The size of systematic error that causes a 5% maximum defect rate for the analytical process. Calculated as $[(TE_a - bias)/s] - 1.65$, where TE_a is the total error specification, and bias is the inaccuracy and s the imprecision (standard deviation) of the measurement procedure.

Cumulative sum control procedure, cusum. A type of control procedure where the differences between control measurements and a target value—usually the established mean for the control material—are calculated and added together successively to provide the cumulative sum of the differences, which is the control statistic that is plotted and interpreted. Two different techniques are in use, "V-mask" cusum, where interpretation depends on the angle of the plotted line, and "decision limit" cusum, where interpretation depends on comparing the cusum with a numerical limit.

Defect. "A departure of a quality characteristic from its intended level or state that occurs with a severity sufficient to cause an associated product or service not to satisfy intended normal, or reasonably foreseeable, usage requirements" (ASQC). When used with reference to the performance of an analytical process, a defect is a patient's test result having a medically important error.

Defect rate. The portion of patients' test results having medically important errors. The quality of an analytical process is inversely related to its defect rate: i.e., the lower the defect rate, the higher the quality; the higher the defect rate, the lower the quality.

Degrees of freedom, df. The number of independent comparisons that can be made among N observations. It may be thought of as the number of measurements in a set minus the number of restrictions on the set. For example, there are $N - 1$ degrees of freedom for the standard deviation because the mean has been calculated prior to the calculation of the standard deviation.

Dispersion. The spread of values observed for a variable. The standard deviation is a measure of dispersion when the distribution is gaussian, whereas the mean is a measure of central tendency or location.

Distribution. The shape of a frequency curve of some variable. A histogram is one form of displaying a frequency curve graphically. The gaussian curve is one type of a distribution.

Electronic spreadsheet. A computer program, such as Lotus 1-2-3, Multi-Plan, etc., that provides a worksheet format of rows and columns, like an accounting form. Equations can be stored in the cells of the worksheet and calculations are automatically performed once data are entered.

Error. See Analytical error.

External quality control. "The procedure of utilizing, for control purposes, the results of several laboratories which analyze the same specimen(s)" (IFCC).

Failure-costs, F-costs. That portion of quality-costs that are incurred because of producing a product with unsatisfactory quality. Internal failure-costs occur when a laboratory repeats analytical runs that are out of control; external failure-costs occur when incorrect analytical results are reported, causing repeat requests and additional testing.

False accept run. An analytical run with errors that is incorrectly accepted by the control procedure.

False reject run. An analytical run without errors that is incorrectly rejected by the control procedure.

Frequency of errors, frequency of occurrence of analytical errors, f. A performance characteristic of a measurement procedure that describes how frequently analytical errors are expected to occur. Related to the stability of the measurement procedure.

Gaussian curve, gaussian distribution, normal curve, normal distribution. A symmetrical bell-shaped distribution whose shape is given by a specific mathematical equation (called the normal equation) in which the mean and standard deviation are variables. It is commonly assumed that the random error of an analytical process fits a gaussian distribution and can therefore be characterized by the standard deviation. The standard deviation is not a valid statistic when the distributions are not gaussian. The terms normal curve and normal distribution are popular in the statistical literature, but are confusing in the clinical literature because of the use of "normal range" for describing the distribution of values for a healthy population.

Imprecision. "Standard deviation or coefficient of variation of the results in a set of replicate measurements. The mean value and number of replicates must be stated, and the design used must be described in such a way that other workers can repeat it. This is particularly important whenever a specific term is used to denote a particular type of imprecision, such as between-laboratory, within-day, or between day" (IFCC).

Inaccuracy. "Numerical difference between the mean of a set of replicate measurements and the true value. This difference (positive or negative) may be expressed in the units in which the quantity is measured, or as a percentage of the true value" (IFCC). Note that this definition implies a systematic error concept of accuracy. More broadly, inaccuracy can be defined as the numerical difference between a measurement and the true value, including both random and systematic components of error (a total error concept of accuracy).

Individual-value control chart. A control chart on which individual control measurements are plotted directly, without any prior calculations having been performed.

Inherent imprecision, inherent random error. The standard deviation or coefficient of variation of the results in a set of replicate measurements when the measurement procedure is operating under stable conditions.

Intermittent analytical errors. Analytical errors that occur in an individual run, but not necessarily in the following runs; the errors are independent from one run to another and do not persist.

Internal quality control. "Procedure of utilizing the results of only one laboratory for quality control purposes" (IFCC).

Just-in-time process, JIT. A production process where a component is produced or delivered just in time for use to avoid maintaining an inventory. The JIT concept is important because a JIT process depends on quality. Delivery of health care can be considered a JIT process.

Levey–Jennings control chart. A commonly used control procedure in which control measurements are plotted directly on a control chart with limit lines drawn either as $\bar{x} \pm 2s$ or $\bar{x} \pm 3s$.

Mean, $\bar{x}$. The arithmetic average of a set of values. Calculated from the equation $\bar{x} = \Sigma x_i/n$, where x_i is an individual measurement and n is the number of measurements. The mean is a measure of the central tendency of a distribution, and, when used in describing analytical processes, is usually related to accuracy. The standard deviation of the distribution is a measure of its width or dispersion and, when used in describing analytical processes, is usually related to precision.

Measurement procedure. The protocol, materials, and equipment necessary for an analyst to obtain a measurement of a patient's sample. It is that part of an analytical process that is concerned with obtaining a measurement, but it does not include assessing the quality of the measurement.

Medical decision level, decision level, X_c. A concentration of analyte where medical interpretation is critical for patient care. There may be several different medical decision levels for a particular analyte.

Medically important errors. Those errors that, when added to the inherent imprecision and inaccuracy of a measurement procedure, cause the total error specification to be exceeded. *Medically important random errors* are those increases in the standard deviation of the measurement procedure that cause the error distribution to exceed the total error specification. *Medically important systematic errors* are those shifts in the mean of the error distribution that cause the error distribution to exceed the total error specification.

Medical usefulness. The concept that the requirements for the performance of an analytical process depend on how the analytical results are used and interpreted medically.

Method evaluation. The process of testing a measurement procedure to evaluate its performance. The magnitudes of the analytical errors are experimentally determined and their acceptability for the application of the method is assessed.

Model. A mathematical equation that describes the behavior of a process as a function of its important characteristics.

Multi-rule quality-control procedure. A control procedure that uses two or more control rules for testing control measurements and determining control status. At least one rule is chosen for its ability to detect random errors and one to detect systematic errors.

Multi-stage quality-control procedure. A control procedure involving two or more different designs, switching from one to another when appropriate. For example, a multi-stage control procedure could have a "start-up" design that is used for initial testing, a "monitoring" design that is used for routine operation following start-up, and a "retrospective" design that is used to review control data over a period longer than a single run.

Normal curve. See Gaussian curve.

Number of control measurements, N. The number of control measurements available for use in testing the quality of an analytical run.

Pareto principle. The concept that a small number of causes are responsible for a high proportion of the problems.

Performance characteristics. Those properties that describe how well a procedure performs. For a control procedure, the performance characteristics are the probabilities for error detection and false rejection, or the average run lengths for rejectable and acceptable quality. For a measurement procedure, the performance characteristics include analytical range, precision, accuracy, interference, and recovery, but also the frequency and duration of analytical errors.

Persistent analytical errors. Analytical errors that, once they occur, are present in the following runs until detected and removed; the errors are not independent from one run to another.

Planning models. The mathematical equations or models that are used to predict the "defect rate" (quality) and "test yield" (productivity) of an analytical process, and therefore aid in planning cost-effective control procedures.

Power curve. "The curve showing the relation between the probability $(1 - \beta)$ of rejecting the hypothesis that a sample belongs to a given population with a given characteristic(s) and the actual population value of that characteristic(s). If β, the probability of accepting the hypothesis, is used instead of $(1 - \beta)$, the curve is called an operating characteristic (OC) curve" (ASQC).

Power-function graph. A graphical presentation of the performance characteristics of a control procedure, such that the probability for rejection is plotted on the y-axis vs the size of error on the x-axis. The probability for false rejection can be read from the y-intercept of a power curve. The probability for error detection can be found by first selecting the size of error on the x-axis, drawing a line up to intersect the power curve, then reading the probability for rejection across on the y-axis. Two power-function graphs are necessary to describe the performance of a control procedure, one for random error and one for systematic error.

Precision. "The agreement between replicate measurements. It has no numerical value" (IFCC, NCCLS). See also Imprecision.

Predictive value characteristics. Secondary features or characteristics of an analytical process that describe the combined effects of the measurement and control procedures and the expected behavior of the resulting analytical process.

Predictive value of an accept signal, PV_a. A characteristic of an analytical process that describes what portion of the accept signals are true accepts.

Predictive value of a reject signal, PV_r. A characteristic of an analytical process that describes what portion of the reject signals are true rejects.

Predictive value of both reject and accept signals, $PV_{r\&a}$. A characteristic of an analytical process that describes what portion of all control signals are true rejects and true accepts.

Prevention-costs, P-costs. That portion of quality-costs that are incurred to prevent defects, or errors, from occurring.

Probability, P. The likelihood that an event will occur. It is usually stated as a decimal fraction between 0 and 1, 0 meaning that the event will never occur, and 1 meaning the event will always occur. For example, P = 0.05 means a probability of 5% that the event will occur.

Probability for rejection, *P*. The probability that a control procedure will give a rejection signal. A probability for rejection of 1.00 means that a rejection always occurs, whereas a probability of 0.00 means that a rejection never occurs.

Probability for error detection, P_{ed}. A performance characteristic of a control procedure that describes the probability of rejecting an analytical run when its results contain errors in addition to the inherent imprecision of the measurement procedure. Ideally, P_{ed} should be 1.00.

Probability for false rejection, P_{fr}. A performance characteristic of a control procedure that describes the probability of rejecting an analytical run when there are no errors in its results except for the inherent imprecision of the measurement procedure. Ideally, P_{fr} should be 0.00.

Productivity. A ratio of output to input for a process. The "test yield" of an analytical process is a measure of its productivity because it describes what portion of analytical tests performed produce correct patients' results.

Project team. A small group of people appointed by management to solve a specific quality problem.

Proportional systematic error. An error that is always in one direction and whose magnitude is a percentage of the concentration of analyte being measured.

Quality. "The totality of features and characteristics of a product or service that bear on its ability to satisfy given needs" (ASQC). When used here, quality means conformance to the requirements of a user or customer, who is generally a physician or nurse acting on behalf of a patient.

Quality assurance. "All those planned or systematic actions necessary to provide adequate confidence that a product or service will satisfy given needs" (ASQC).

Quality circle. A group of people who voluntarily meet regularly to identify and solve quality-related problems, including quality of work life issues.

Quality control. "The study of those errors which are the responsibility of the laboratory, and the procedures used to recognize and minimize them. This study includes all errors arising within the laboratory between the receipt of the specimen and the dispatch of the report. On some occasions, the responsibility of the laboratory may extend to the collection of the specimen from the patient, and the provision of a suitable container" (IFCC).

Quality-costs, Q-costs. The costs associated with producing a product or service, in this case a test result, with the quality necessary to satisfy the user or customer, as well as the costs incurred from products and services of unsatisfactory quality. Composed of prevention-costs, appraisal-costs, and failure-costs.

Quality-costs model. A mathematical equation that describes quality-costs as a function of the characteristics of a process, in this case an analytical process, and permits those costs to be predicted from the error-detection and false-rejection characteristics of the control procedure and from the frequency of errors of the measurement procedure.

Quality management. A management approach that places quality first in importance in management activities and decision making. Other names applied to this same approach include "quality improvement" and "total quality control." More narrowly defined by ASQC to mean "the totality of functions involved in the determination and achievement of quality."

Quality–productivity planning model. A model that predicts the quality ("defect rate") and productivity ("test yield") of an analytical process, as a function of the control procedure's error-detection and false-rejection characteristics and the measurement procedure's frequency of errors. Derived from a quality-costs model by interpreting cost in terms of the costs of repeat runs and repeat requests. Useful for planning purposes to study the effects of different designs of quality control on the cost-effectiveness of the analytical process.

Quality requirements. The many features and characteristics of a laboratory testing service that bear on its ability to satisfy its users or customers.

Random access analytical process. A type of analytical process that is calibrated, tested for control, then used for analysis of patients' specimens. Instrument systems with long-term stability are often operated this way and tested for control only periodically.

Random analytical error. An error that can be either positive or negative, the direction and exact magnitude of which cannot be predicted. In contrast, systematic errors are always in one direction.

R-chart, range chart. A type of control chart in which the range, or difference between the high and low values in a group of N control measurements, is plotted vs time (or run number). It is primarily sensitive to random error or imprecision, in contrast to an $\bar{x}$-chart ("x-bar" or mean), which is sensitive to systematic error or inaccuracy. Range and mean charts are usually used together.

Response curve. A plot of the probability of rejection (for a specified error condition) of a control rule vs the number of control measurements (N).

Result. "Final value obtained for a measured quantity after performing a measuring procedure including all subprocedures and laboratory evaluation" (IFCC). Laboratory evaluation here would be interpreted as any and all quality-control evaluations; thus, the result is the final value obtained from an analytical process.

Sample. "The appropriate representative part of a specimen which is used in the analysis" (IFCC).

S-chart, standard deviation chart. A type of control chart in which the standard deviation of a group of N control measurements is plotted vs time (or run number) to monitor random error or imprecision. Generally replaced by a range chart when N <10 per run.

Sensitivity. See Chemical sensitivity, Clinical sensitivity.

Simultaneous batch process. An analytical process wherein calibrators, controls, and patients' samples are analyzed for several different analytes at the same time. Several batch processes are run in parallel.

Specificity. See Chemical specificity, Clinical specificity.

Specimen. "Material available for analysis" (IFCC).

Standard deviation, s. A statistic that describes the dispersion or spread of a set of measurements about the mean value. Calculated from the equation:

$$s = \sqrt{[n\Sigma x_i^2 - (\Sigma x_i)^2]/[n(n-1)]}$$

where n is the number of measurements, and x_i is an individual measurement.

State of statistical control. "A process is considered to be in a 'state of statistical control' if the variations among the observed sampling results from it can be attributed to a constant system of chance causes" (ASQC).

Statistical quality control. Those aspects of quality control in which statistics are applied, in contrast to other aspects in which statistics are not required. Statistical procedures are most often used to monitor a measurement procedure and alert the analyst to changes in performance. Control charts are statistical procedures.

Systematic analytical error. An error that is always in one direction, in contrast to random errors that may be either positive or negative and whose direction cannot be predicted.

Test of significance. A statistical test to determine whether the experimental data are sufficient to support a conclusion that there is a difference between two quantities. Control rules are statistical tests used to determine whether the mean and standard deviation of an analytical process have changed from their original, stable values. Mean and chi-square control rules are tests of significance for the mean and standard deviation, respectively.

Test yield. The portion of measurements from an analytical process that are correct and reportable as patients' results. Test yield provides a measure of the productivity of an analytical process in terms of test utilization.

Total error. The net or combined effect of the random and systematic errors.

Total error specification, allowable total error, TE_a. The total amount of analytical error that can be tolerated without invalidating the medical usefulness of the analytical result. TE_a can be used to decide the acceptability of a measurement procedure in method evaluation testing, or to calculate the size of medically important errors to aid in the selection or design of control procedures. When applied to method evaluation testing, we recommend that TE_a be used as a 99% limit of error so that only 1 sample in 100 will have a greater amount of error; this allows a defect rate of 1% when the analytical process is under stable operation. When applied as a quality specification for the selection or design of control procedures, we recommend that TE_a be used as a 95% limit of errors, implying a maximum defect rate of 5% when the process experiences unstable operation.

True accept run. An analytical run without errors that is correctly accepted by the control procedure.

True reject run. An analytical run with errors that is correctly rejected by the control procedure.

True value. Generally taken to mean the correct value for a parameter, such as the correct analytical concentration for a specimen.

Type I error. "The incorrect decision that a process is unacceptable when, in fact, perfect information would reveal that it is within the 'zone of acceptable processes' " (ASQC).

Type II error. The incorrect decision that a process is acceptable when, in fact, perfect information would reveal that it is located within the 'zone of rejectable processes' " (ASQC).

Variable. A quantity of interest, the value or magnitude of which fluctuates or changes.

Variance, s^2. The standard deviation squared. When sources of error are independent of each other, the variance of the total error is the sum of the variances due to the individual sources of error. Useful for calculating appropriate control limits when there are both within-run and between-run components of variance.

Warning limits. "Limits at which attention is called to the possibility of out-of-control conditions, but further action is not necessarily required. (When warning limits, which are usually located inside the control limits, are used, the regular control limits are often called action limits.)" (ASQC).

Westgard rules, Westgard multi-rule control procedure. A control procedure that uses a series of control rules to test the control measurements. A 1_{2s} rule is used as a warning, followed by use of 1_{3s}, 2_{2s}, R_{4s}, 4_{1s}, and $10_{\bar{x}}$ as rejection rules. See Chapter 4 for a detailed discussion, including example interpretations of control data. See Glossary of Control Rules for definitions of abbreviations or symbols.

Within-run standard deviation, within-run component of variation, s_w. The standard deviation calculated from replicate measurements within a single analytical run. It describes the short-term precision or random error occurring in a single run, in contrast to the between-run standard deviation, s_b, which describes the precision or random error of a series of averages (of several replicates within a run) determined in different analytical runs.

$\bar{x}$-chart, "x-bar" or mean chart. A type of control chart in which the mean of a group of N control measurements is plotted vs time (or run number). Primarily sensitive to systematic error or inaccuracy, in contrast to the range chart, which is sensitive to random error or imprecision. Mean and range charts are usually used together.

Zero defects. Refers to the concept that no mistakes or errors are allowable. Particularly important as a goal in health care because of the potentially serious consequences of an individual mistake or error.

References

ASQC. Glossary and tables for statistical quality control. Milwaukee, WI: American Society for Quality Control, 1983.

IFCC. Buttner J, Borth R, Boutwell JH, Broughton PMG. International Federation of Clinical Chemistry provisional recommendation on quality control in clinical chemistry. I. General principles and terminology. Clin Chem 1976; 22:532–40.

NCCLS. Document C24-P, Internal quality control testing: principles and definitions; proposed guidelines. Villanova, PA: National Committee for Clinical Laboratory Standards, 1985.

Glossary of Control Rules

Many different criteria can be used to interpret control data. We use the term *control rule* to represent a decision criterion by which one interprets control data and makes a judgment on the control status of an analytical run. We use symbols of the general form A_L, where A is the abbreviation for a paticular statistic or is the number of control measurements, and L is the control limit. An analytical run is rejected when the control measurements fulfill the stated conditions, i.e., when a certain statistic or number of control measurements exceeds specified limits.

Control rules can be applied *within a material* to test the measurements of a single control material collected within a single analytical run; *within a material, across runs* to test the measurements of a single control material collected from more than one analytical run; *across materials* to test the measurements of two or more control materials collected within a single analytical run; *across materials, across runs* to test the measurements of two or more control materials collected in two or more analytical runs.

$\mathbf{1_{2s}}$. One control measurement exceeds $\bar{x} \pm 2s$. Historically, this was a "warning" limit on a Shewhart chart, but it is more often used in clinical laboratories as a rejection limit on a Levey–Jennings chart.

$\mathbf{1_{3s}}$. One control measurement exceeds $\bar{x} \pm 3s$. This is the "action" or rejection limit recommended for a Shewhart control chart, and is similarly used on Levey–Jennings charts in clinical laboratories.

$\mathbf{2_{2s}}$. Two consecutive control measurements exceed the same limit, which is either $\bar{x} + 2s$ or $\bar{x} - 2s$.

$\mathbf{R_{4s}}$. The difference between the high and low control measurements within a run exceeds 4s.

$\mathbf{3_{1s}}$. Three consecutive control measurements exceed the same limit, which is either $\bar{x} + 1s$ or $\bar{x} - 1s$.

$\mathbf{4_{1s}}$. Four consecutive control measurements exceed the same limit, which is either $\bar{x} + 1s$ or $\bar{x} - 1s$.

$\mathbf{7_{\bar{x}}}$. Seven consecutive control measurements fall on one side of the mean.

$\mathbf{7_T}$. Seven consecutive control measurements show a trend upwards, or downwards.

$10_{\bar{x}}$. Ten consecutive control measurements fall on one side of the mean.

$1_{P_{fr}}$. One control measurement in a group of N control measurements exceeds control limits that have been chosen to have a specified probability for false rejection, P_{fr}. For example, $1_{0.05}$ would be a control rule having limits chosen to maintain a 0.05 probability for false rejection. The control limits change with N, widening as N increases (see Table AI-2 in Appendix I for factors for calculating the control limits).

$2_{P_{fr}}$. Two consecutive control measurements in a group of N control measurements exceed the same control limit, which is chosen to have a specified probability for false rejection, P_{fr}. For example, $2_{0.05}$ is a control rule having limits chosen to maintain a 0.05 probability for false rejection. The control limits change with N, widening as N increases (see Table AI-2 in Appendix I).

CS. The differences between the individual control measurements and $\bar{x}$ are calculated and summed to give the total or cumulative sum. The "cusum" is then judged by graphical techniques—V-mask cusum—or by numerical control limits—decision limit cusum.

$\bar{x}_{P_{fr}}$. The mean of a group of N control measurements exceeds control limits having a specified probability for false rejection, P_{fr}. For example, $\bar{x}_{0.05}$ would be a "mean rule" with control limits chosen to maintain a 0.05 probability of false rejection. The actual limits decrease as N increases, so as to keep P_{fr} constant (see Table AI-2, Appendix I).

$R_{P_{fr}}$. The range, or difference between the high and low measurements in a group of N control measurements, exceeds an upper one-sided control limit having a specified probability for false rejection, P_{fr}. For example, $R_{0.05}$ would be a "range rule" with control limits chosen to maintain a 0.05 probability of false rejection. The actual control limits increase as N increases, so as to keep P_{fr} constant (see Table AI-2 in Appendix I).

$\chi^2_{P_{fr}}$. The ratio $s^2_{obs}\ (N - 1)/s^2$ exceeds the critical chi-square value having a specified P_{fr}, where s_{obs} is the standard deviation observed (or calculated) from the control measurements and s is the stable standard deviation of the measurement procedure. For example, $\chi^2_{0.05}$ is a "chi-square rule" with control limits chosen to maintain a 0.05 probability of false rejection. The critical chi-square value varies with N and with the chosen P_{fr} (see Table AI-2 in Appendix I).

APPENDIX I

Statistical Tables

Table AI-1. Areas under the Upper Tail of a Gaussian Curve[a]

	s									
s	.00	.01	.02	.03	.04	.05	.06	.07	.08	.09
0.0	.5000	.4960	.4920	.4880	.4840	.4801	.4761	.4721	.4681	.4641
0.1	.4602	.4562	.4522	.4483	.4443	.4404	.4364	.4325	.4286	.4247
0.2	.4207	.4168	.4129	.4090	.4052	.4013	.3974	.3936	.3897	.3859
0.3	.3821	.3783	.3745	.3707	.3669	.3632	.3594	.3557	.3520	.3483
0.4	.3446	.3409	.3372	.3336	.3300	.3264	.3228	.3192	.3156	.3121
0.5	.3085	.3050	.3015	.2981	.2946	.2912	.2877	.2843	.2810	.2776
0.6	.2743	.2709	.2676	.2643	.2611	.2578	.2546	.2514	.2483	.2451
0.7	.2420	.2389	.2358	.2327	.2296	.2266	.2236	.2206	.2177	.2148
0.8	.2119	.2090	.2061	.2033	.2005	.1977	.1949	.1922	.1894	.1867
0.9	.1841	.1814	.1788	.1762	.1736	.1711	.1685	.1660	.1635	.1611
1.0	.1587	.1562	.1539	.1515	.1492	.1469	.1446	.1423	.1401	.1379
1.1	.1357	.1335	.1314	.1292	.1271	.1251	.1230	.1210	.1190	.1170
1.2	.1151	.1131	.1112	.1093	.1075	.1056	.1038	.1020	.1003	.0985
1.3	.0968	.0951	.0934	.0918	.0901	.0885	.0869	.0853	.0838	.0823
1.4	.0808	.0793	.0778	.0764	.0749	.0735	.0721	.0708	.0694	.0681
1.5	.0668	.0655	.0643	.0630	.0618	.0606	.0594	.0582	.0571	.0559
1.6	.0548	.0537	.0526	.0516	.0505	.0495	.0485	.0475	.0465	.0455
1.7	.0446	.0436	.0427	.0418	.0409	.0401	.0392	.0384	.0375	.0367
1.8	.0359	.0351	.0344	.0336	.0329	.0322	.0314	.0307	.0301	.0294
1.9	.0287	.0281	.0274	.0268	.0262	.0256	.0250	.0244	.0239	.0233
2.0	.0228	.0222	.0217	.0212	.0207	.0202	.0197	.0192	.0188	.0183

(continued)

Table AI-1. *(continued)*

s	.00	.01	.02	.03	.04	.05	.06	.07	.08	.09
2.1	.0179	.0174	.0170	.0166	.0162	.0158	.0154	.0150	.0146	.0143
2.2	.0139	.0136	.0132	.0129	.0125	.0122	.0119	.0116	.0113	.0110
2.3	.0107	.0104	.0102	.0099	.0096	.0094	.0091	.0089	.0087	.0084
2.4	.0082	.0080	.0078	.0075	.0073	.0071	.0069	.0068	.0066	.0064
2.5	.0062	.0062	.0059	.0057	.0055	.0054	.0052	.0051	.0049	.0048
2.6	.0047	.0045	.0044	.0043	.0041	.0040	.0039	.0038	.0037	.0036
2.7	.0035	.0034	.0033	.0032	.0031	.0030	.0029	.0028	.0027	.0026
2.8	.0026	.0025	.0024	.0023	.0023	.0022	.0021	.0021	.0020	.0019
2.9	.0019	.0018	.0018	.0017	.0016	.0016	.0015	.0015	.0014	.0014
3.0	.0013	.0013	.0013	.0012	.0012	.0011	.0011	.0011	.0010	.0010
3.1	.0010	.0009	.0009	.0009	.0008	.0008	.0008	.0008	.0007	.0007
3.2	.0007	.0007	.0006	.0006	.0006	.0006	.0006	.0005	.0005	.0005
3.3	.0005	.0005	.0005	.0004	.0004	.0004	.0004	.0004	.0004	.0003
3.4	.0003	.0003	.0003	.0003	.0003	.0003	.0003	.0003	.0003	.0002
3.5	.0002	.0002	.0002	.0002	.0002	.0002	.0002	.0002	.0002	.0002

[a] For example, to find the area outside the mean +1.55s, find 1.5 in the left-most column, then read across the row to the column headed 0.05; the value .0606 indicates that 6.06% of the total area under the gaussian curve is found in the upper tail of the curve. Because of the symmetry of the gaussian distribution, 6.06% of the area would also be found in the lower tail (outside the mean −1.55s), for a total of 12.12% outside the mean ±1.55s.

Table AI-2. Factors for Calculating Control Limits

Control rule	N, number of control measurements								
	2	3	4	6	8	10	12	16	20
A. Factors for calculating control limits from the standard deviation									
$1_{0.05}$[a]	2.24	2.39	2.50	2.64	2.74	2.81	2.86	2.94	3.02
$1_{0.01}$	2.81	2.93	3.01	3.13	3.21	3.27	3.31	3.38	3.43
$1_{0.002}$	3.27	3.36	3.44	3.52	3.59	3.64	3.66	3.72	3.75
$2_{0.05}$	1.01	1.22	1.33	1.47	1.56	1.62	1.67	1.74	1.80
$2_{0.01}$	1.47	1.64	1.74	1.86	1.93	2.00	2.03	2.09	2.14
$2_{0.002}$	1.86	2.01	2.09	2.19	2.26	2.30	2.34	2.40	2.44
$\bar{x}_{0.05}$	1.39	1.13	0.98	0.80	0.69	0.62	0.57	0.49	0.44
$\bar{x}_{0.01}$	1.82	1.49	1.29	1.05	0.91	0.82	0.74	0.65	0.58
$\bar{x}_{0.002}$	2.19	1.78	1.54	1.26	1.09	0.98	0.89	0.77	0.69
$R_{0.05}$	2.77	3.31	3.63	4.03	4.29	4.47	4.62	4.85	5.01
$R_{0.01}$	3.64	4.12	4.40	4.76	4.99	5.16	5.29	5.50	5.65
$R_{0.002}$	4.37	4.80	5.05	5.37	5.58	5.75	5.80	6.05	6.20
$s_{0.003}$[b]	1.84	1.86	1.81	1.71	1.64	1.58	1.54	1.48	1.43
B. Factors for calculating control limits from the average range									
$\bar{x}_{0.003}$[c]	1.88	1.02	0.73	0.48	0.37	0.31	0.27	0.21	0.18
$R_{0.003}$	3.27	2.57	2.28	2.00	1.86	1.78	1.72	1.64	1.59
C. Critical values for chi-square test									
$\chi^2_{0.05}$	5.99	7.81	9.49	12.59	15.51	18.31	21.03	26.30	31.41
$\chi^2_{0.01}$	9.21	11.34	13.28	16.81	20.09	23.21	26.22	32.00	37.57
$\chi^2_{0.005}$	10.59	12.83	14.86	18.54	21.95	25.18	28.30	34.26	39.99

[a] From Table 1 in: Westgard JO, Groth T, Aronsson T, Falk H, de Verdier C-H. Performance characteristics of rules for internal quality control: probabilities for false rejection and error detection. Clin Chem 1977;23:1857–67.

[b] From Table E in: Grant EI, Leavenworth RS. Statistical quality control, 5th ed. New York: McGraw Hill, 1980:633.

[c] From Table C: Ibid:631.

APPENDIX II

Power-Function Graphs

Power-function graphs are plots of the probability for rejecting an analytical run (y-axis) vs the size of errors to be detected (x-axis). For random error, the x-axis is labeled ΔRE, the size of random error to be detected, expressed as the factor by which the original stable standard deviation (s) has increased; e.g., a ΔRE of 2.0 indicates that the standard deviation has doubled. For systematic error, the x-axis is labeled ΔSE, the size of systematic error to be detected, given as a multiple of s; e.g., a ΔSE of 2.0s indicates the mean has shifted by an amount equal to two times the stable standard deviation.

The control procedures are indicated by specifying the control rules, using abbreviations of the form A_L. See the Glossary of Control Rules for definitions. The number of control measurements (N) and the number of runs (r) are indicated on the power-function graphs. When errors occur in individual runs, the probability for rejection changes as the rules change and as N changes. When errors persist from run to run and a control procedure utilizes past control data, the probability for rejection also changes with the number of runs.

For random error, a single power-function graph is provided for each control procedure; the different lines on the graph correspond to different values for N. For systematic error, from one to three power-function graphs are provided to describe the effects of both N and r. When only one graph is provided, the different lines represent different values for N; when more than one graph is provided, each graph is for a different N and the lines on each graph are for different values for r. See Chapters 3 and 4 for further discussion and illustrative examples.

These power-function graphs were obtained from computer simulations of 500 to 1000 runs at each error condition. Effects of data rounding and between-run components of variation are not described. Because the graphs were drawn point to point, occasionally visual interpolation will be required to smooth the power curves.

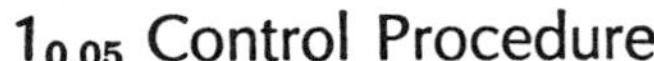

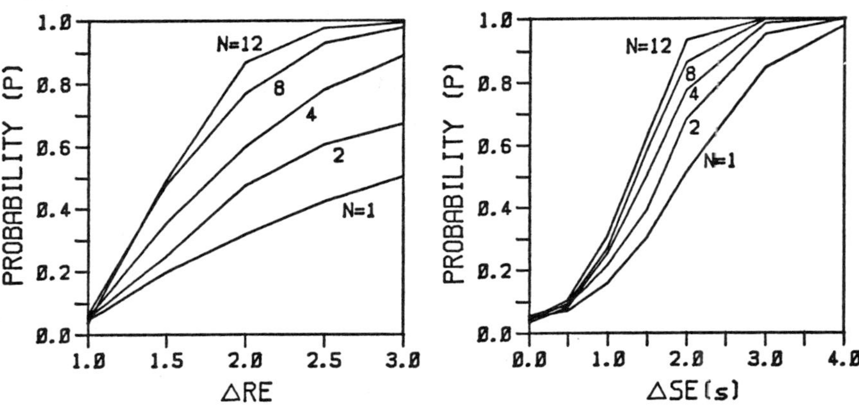

1_{2s} Control Procedure

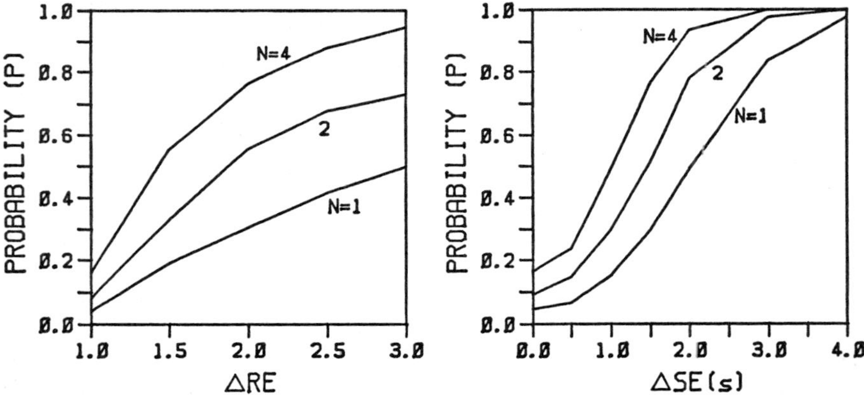

$1_{2s}/4_{1s}$ Control Procedure

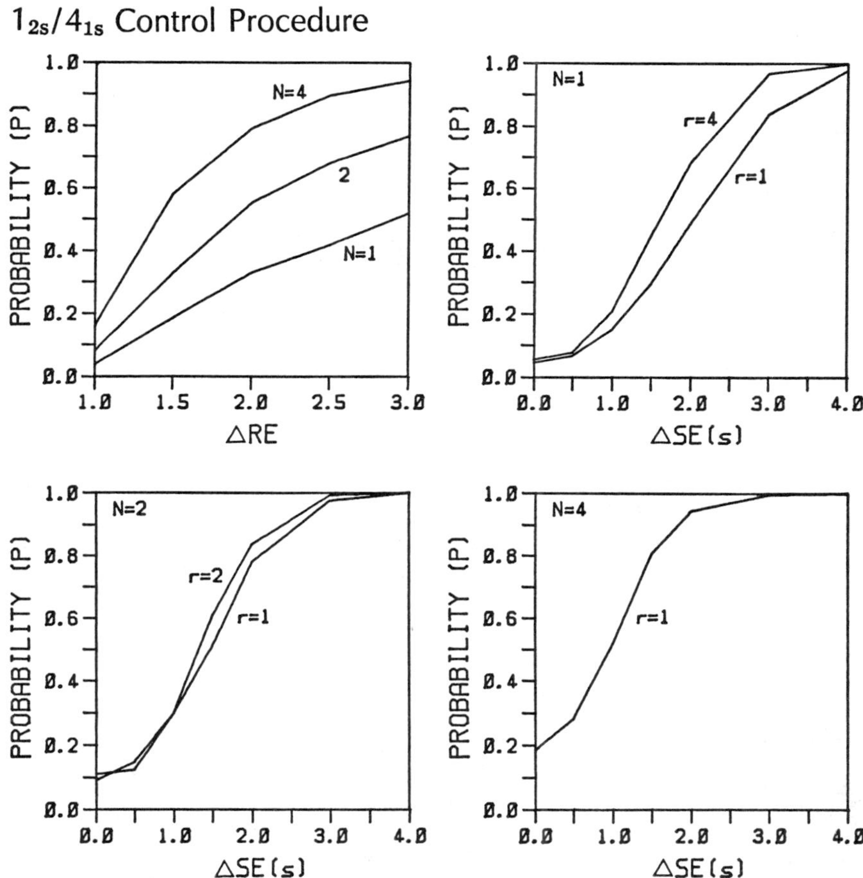

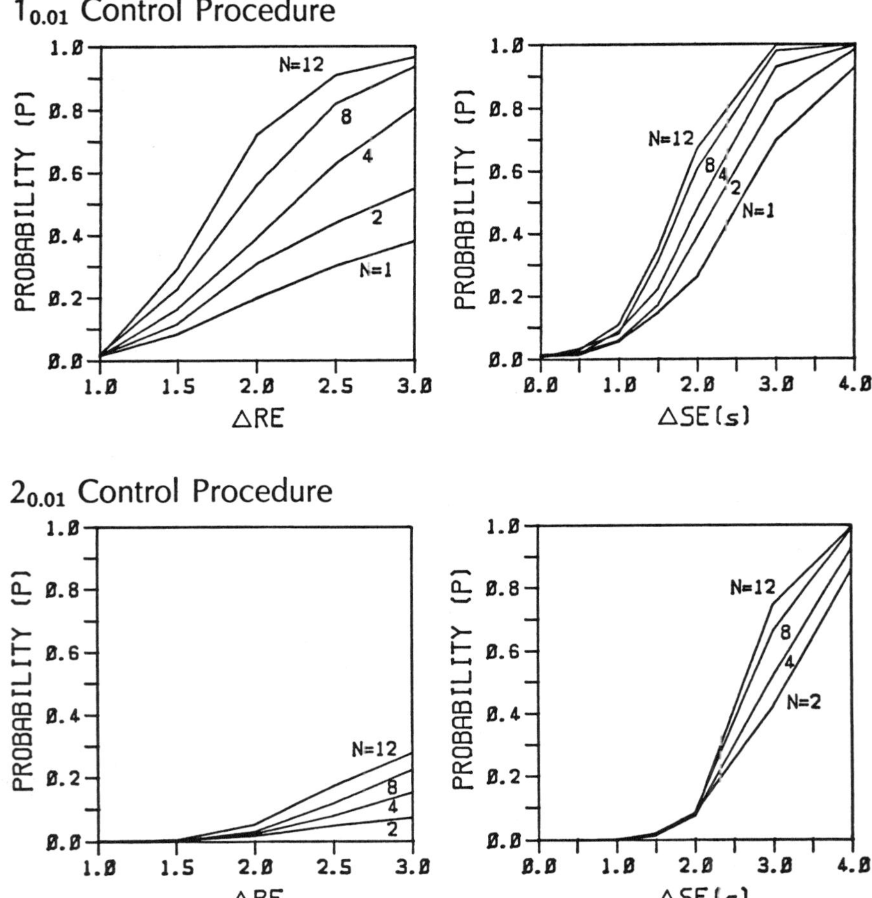

1 0.01 Control Procedure
PROBABILITY (P)
1.0
0.8
0.6
0.4
0.2
0.0
N=12
8
4
2
N=1
1.0
1.5
2.0
2.5
3.0
ΔRE
N=12
8
4
2
N=1
0.0
1.0
2.0
3.0
4.0
ΔSE(s)
2 0.01 Control Procedure
PROBABILITY (P)
N=12
8
4
2
ΔRE
N=12
8
4
N=2
ΔSE(s)

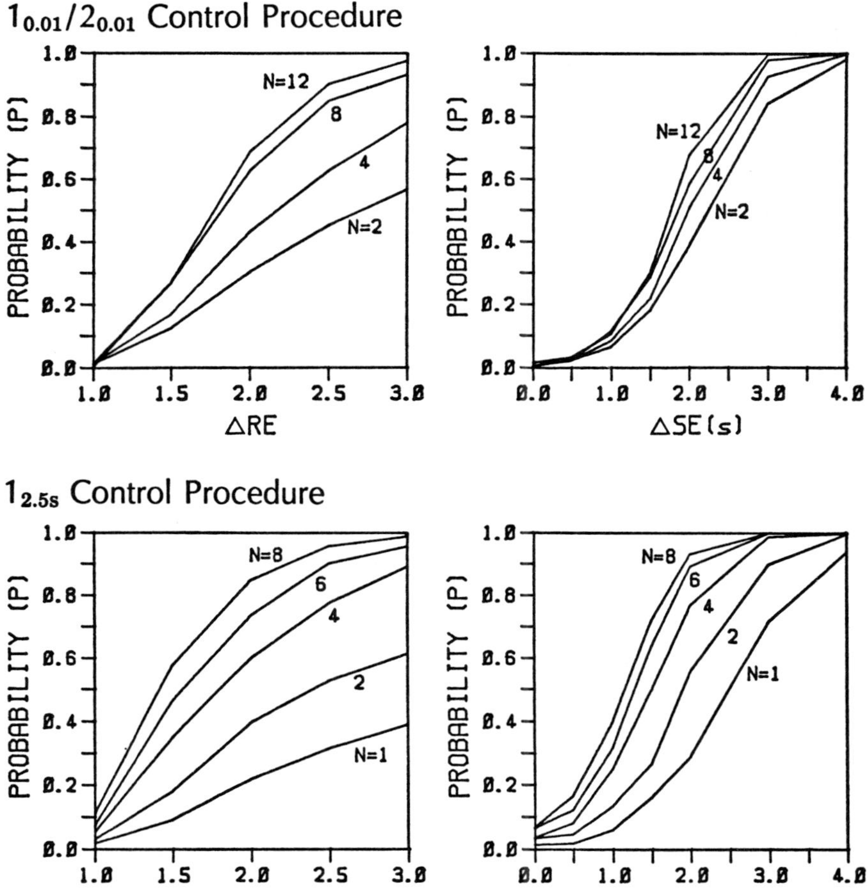
$1_{0.01}/2_{0.01}$ Control Procedure
PROBABILITY (P)
0.0
0.2
0.4
0.6
0.8
1.0
N=12
8
4
N=2
1.0
1.5
2.0
2.5
3.0
ΔRE
PROBABILITY (P)
N=12
8
4
N=2
0.0
1.0
2.0
3.0
4.0
ΔSE(s)
$1_{2.5s}$ Control Procedure
PROBABILITY (P)
N=8
6
4
2
N=1
ΔRE
PROBABILITY (P)
N=8
6
4
2
N=1
ΔSE(s)

$1_{2.5s}/2_{2s}$ Control Procedure

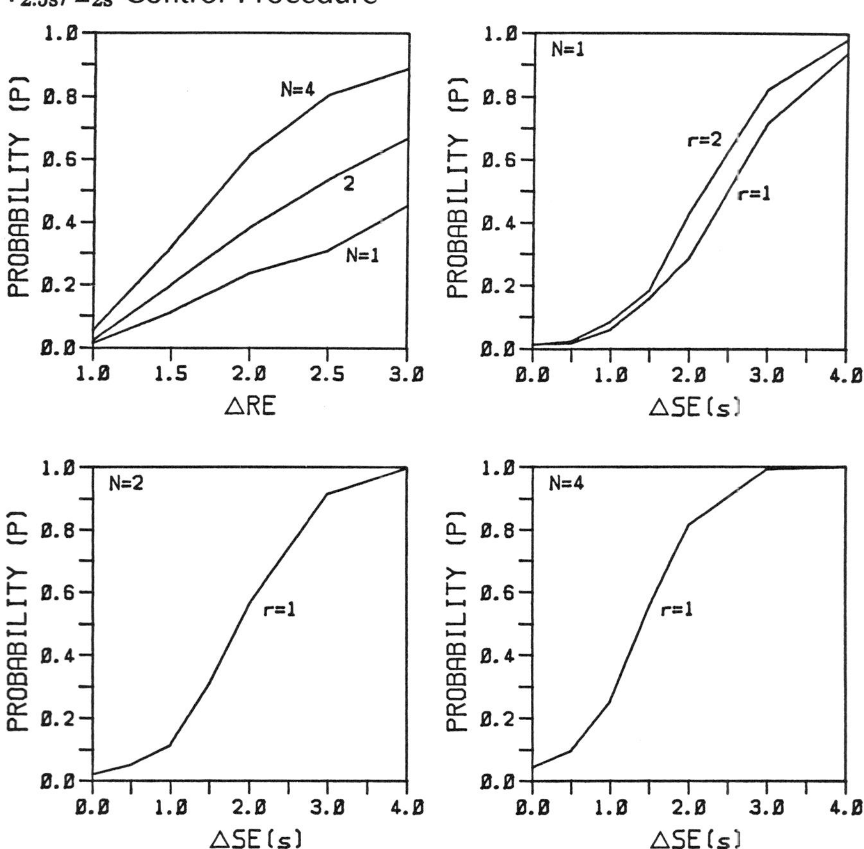

$1_{2.5s}/2_{2s}/R_{4s}$ Control Procedure

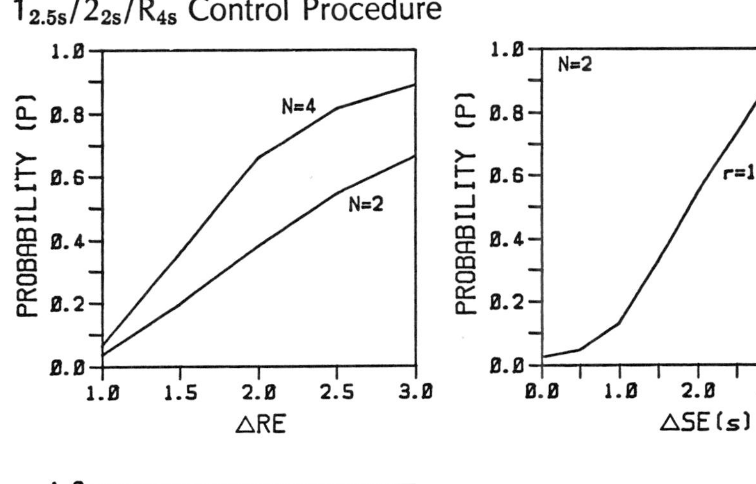

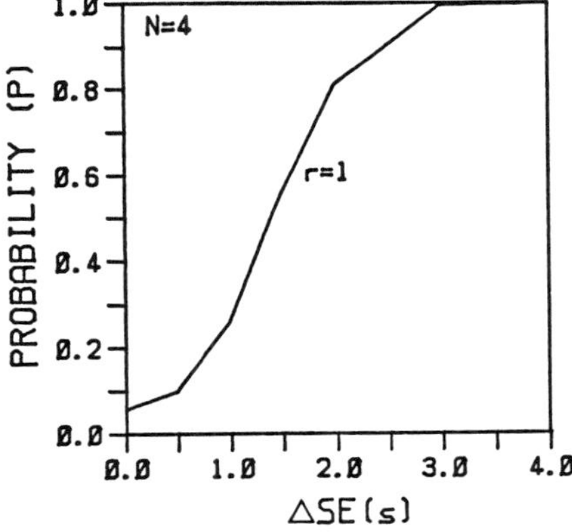

$1_{2.5s}/2_{2s}/4_{1s}$ Control Procedure

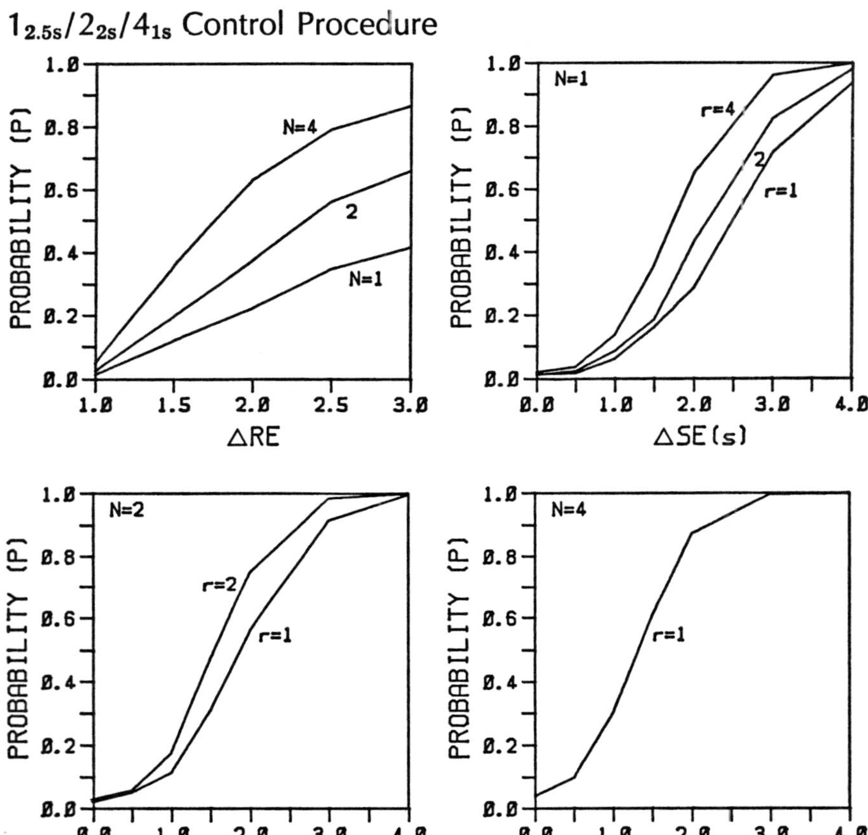

$1_{2.5s}/2_{2s}/R_{4s}/4_{1s}$ Control Procedure

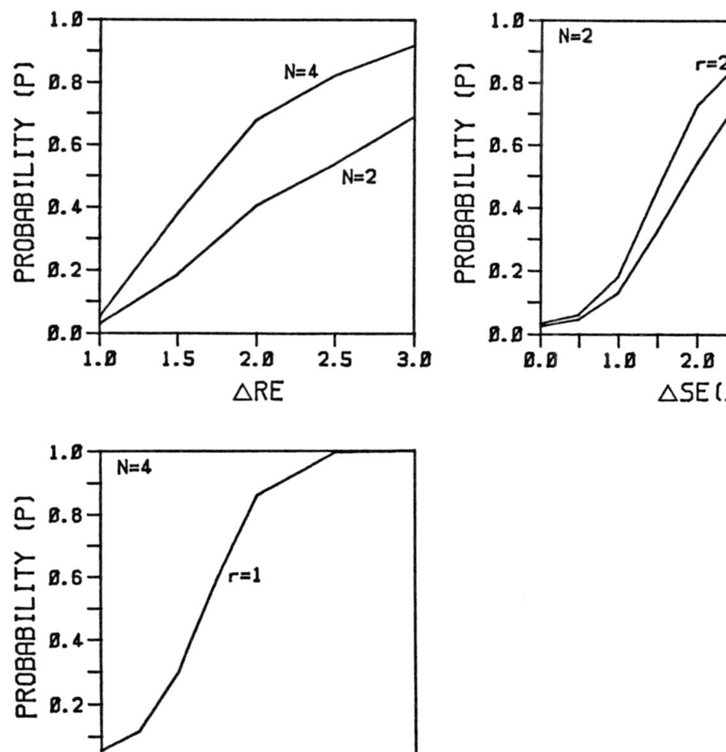

$1_{0.002}$ Control Procedure

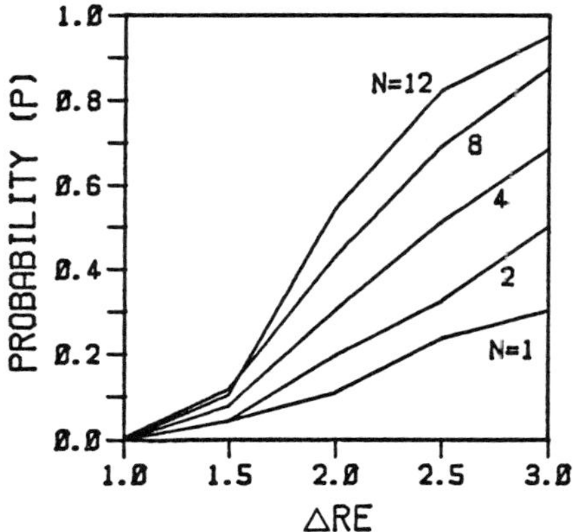

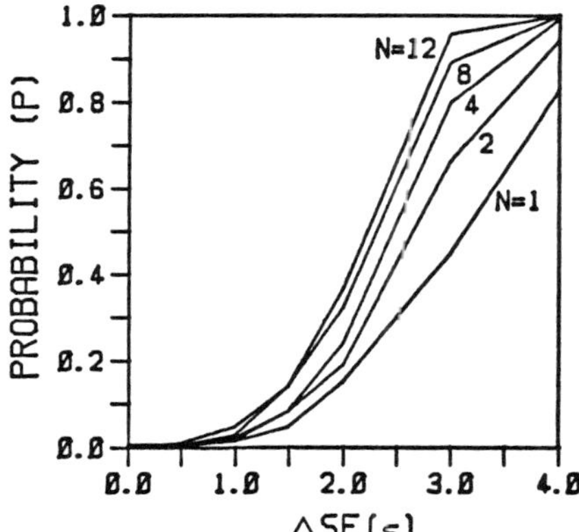

1_{3s} Control Procedure

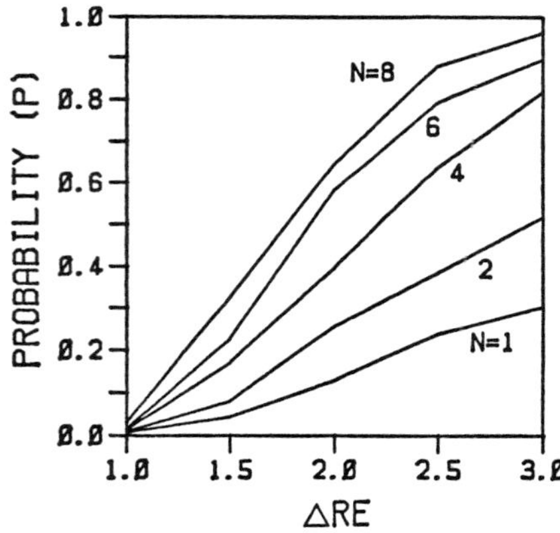

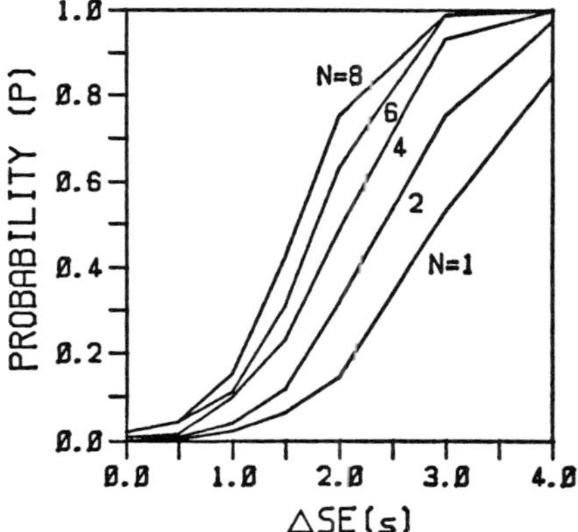

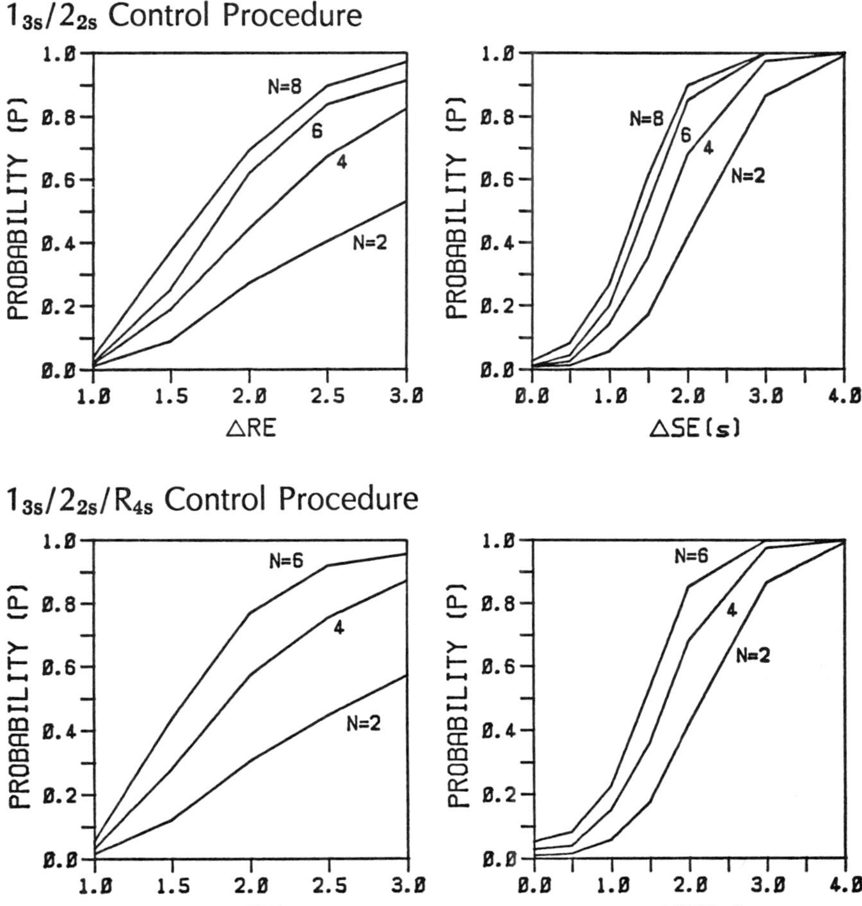

$1_{3s}/2_{2s}$ Control Procedure
PROBABILITY (P)
1.0
0.8
0.6
0.4
0.2
0.0
1.0 1.5 2.0 2.5 3.0
ΔRE
N=8
6
4
N=2
PROBABILITY (P)
0.0 1.0 2.0 3.0 4.0
ΔSE(s)
$1_{3s}/2_{2s}/R_{4s}$ Control Procedure
N=6
4
N=2

$1_{3s}/2_{2s}/R_{4s}/4_{1s}$ Control Procedure

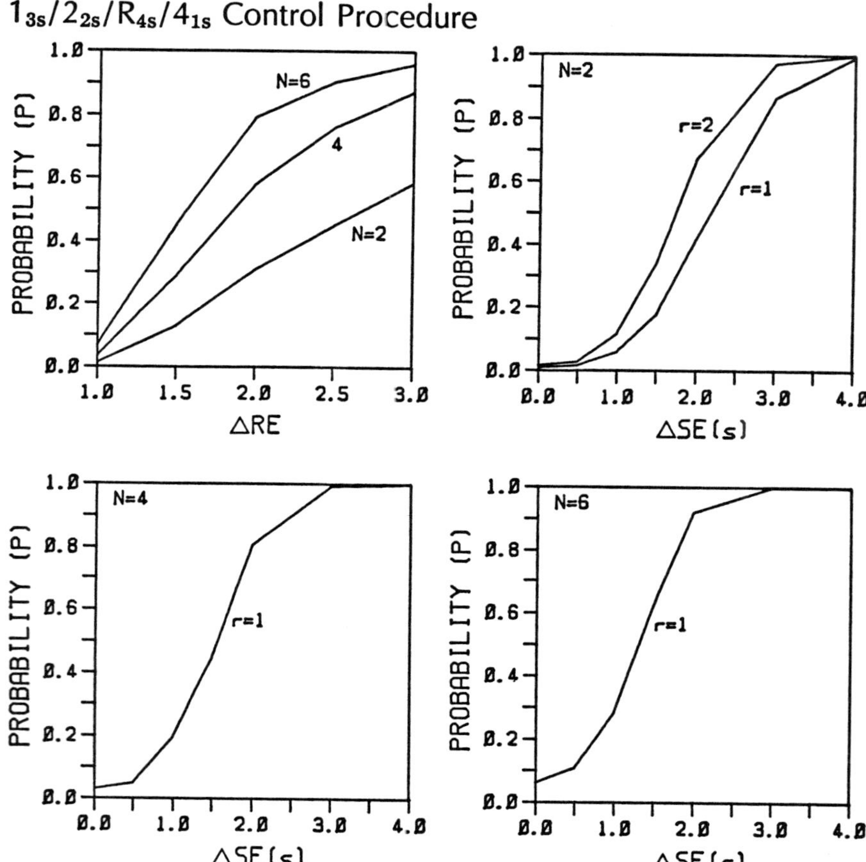

$1_{3s}/2_{2s}/R_{4s}/4_{1s}/10_{\bar{x}}$ Control Procedure

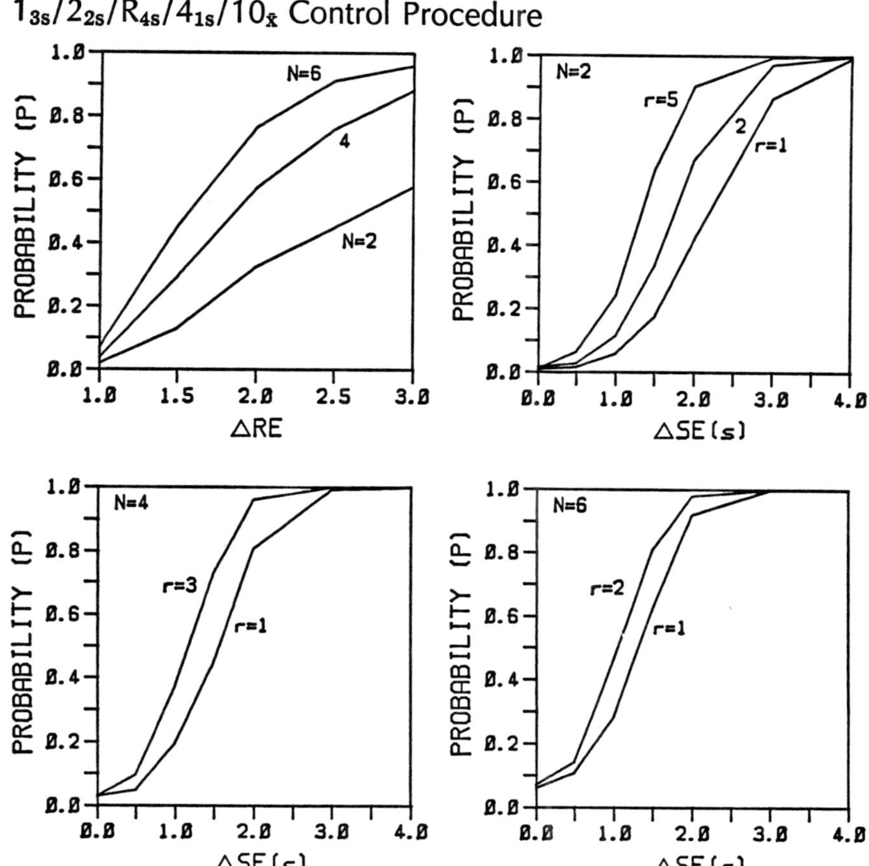

$1_{3s}/2_{2s}/R_{4s}/4_{1s}/8_{\bar{x}}$ Control Procedure

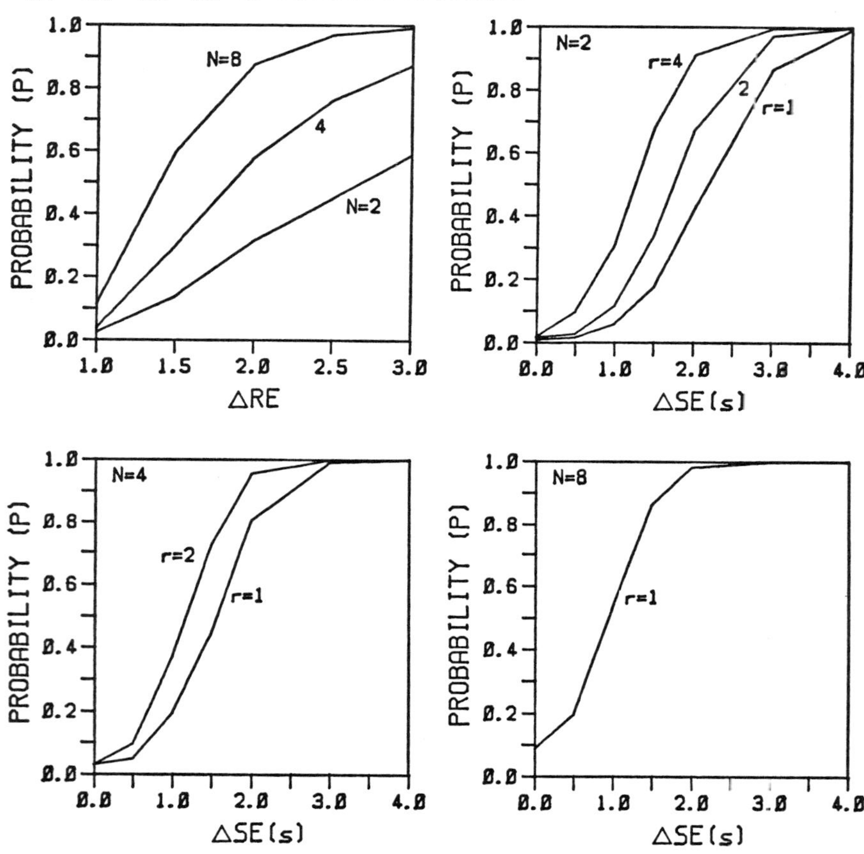

$1_{3s}/2_{2s}/R_{4s}/4_{1s}/12_{\bar{x}}$ Control Procedure

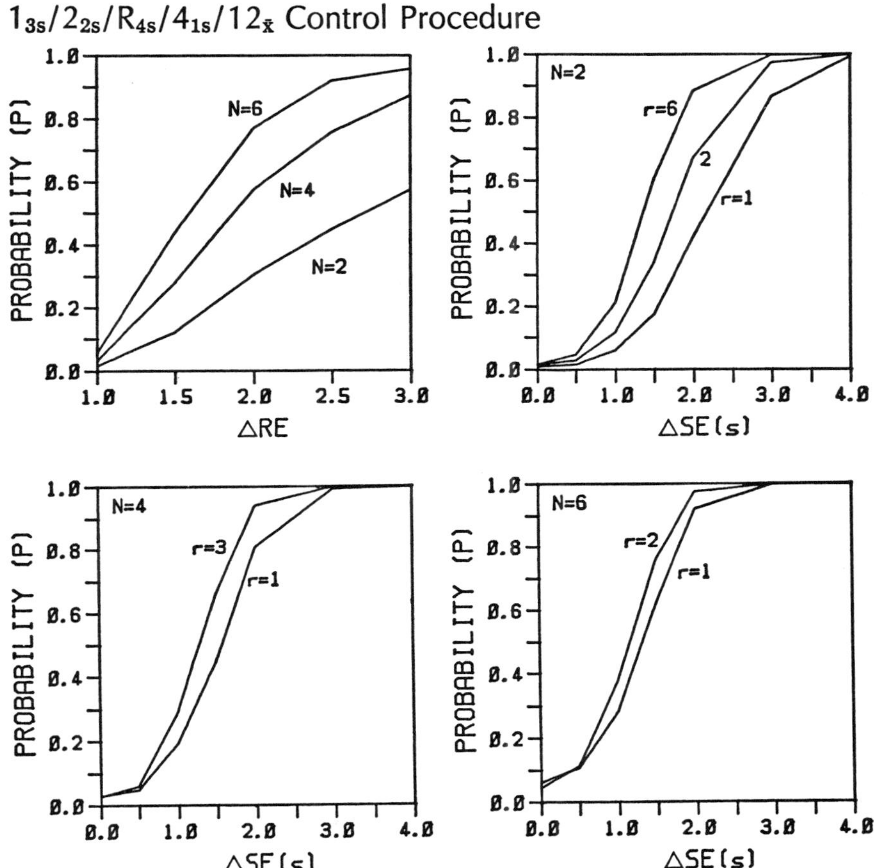

$1_{3s}/(2 \text{ of } 3)_{2s}$ Control Procedure

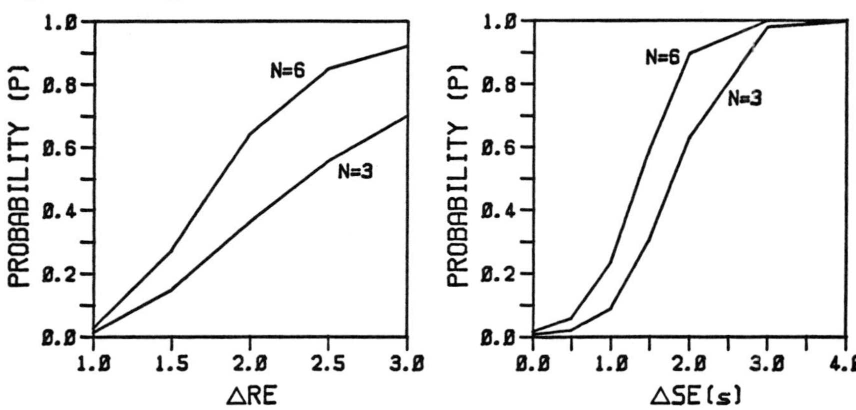

$1_{3s}/(2 \text{ of } 3)_{2s}/R_{4s}$ Control Procedure

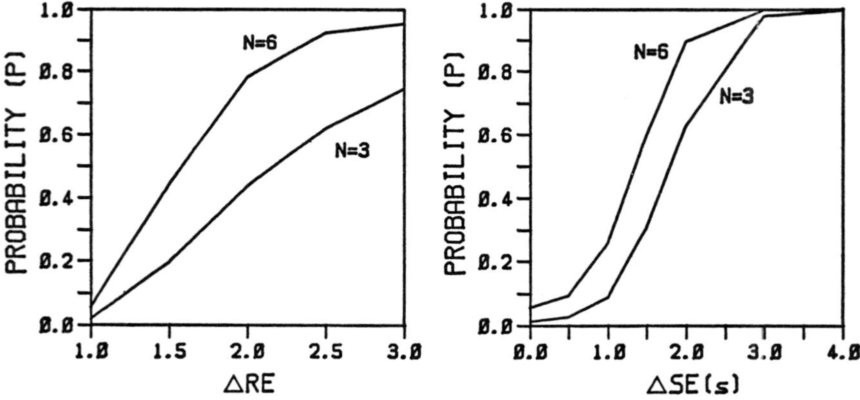

1_{3s} /(2 of 3)$_{2s}$/R$_{4s}$/9$_{\bar{x}}$ Control Procedure

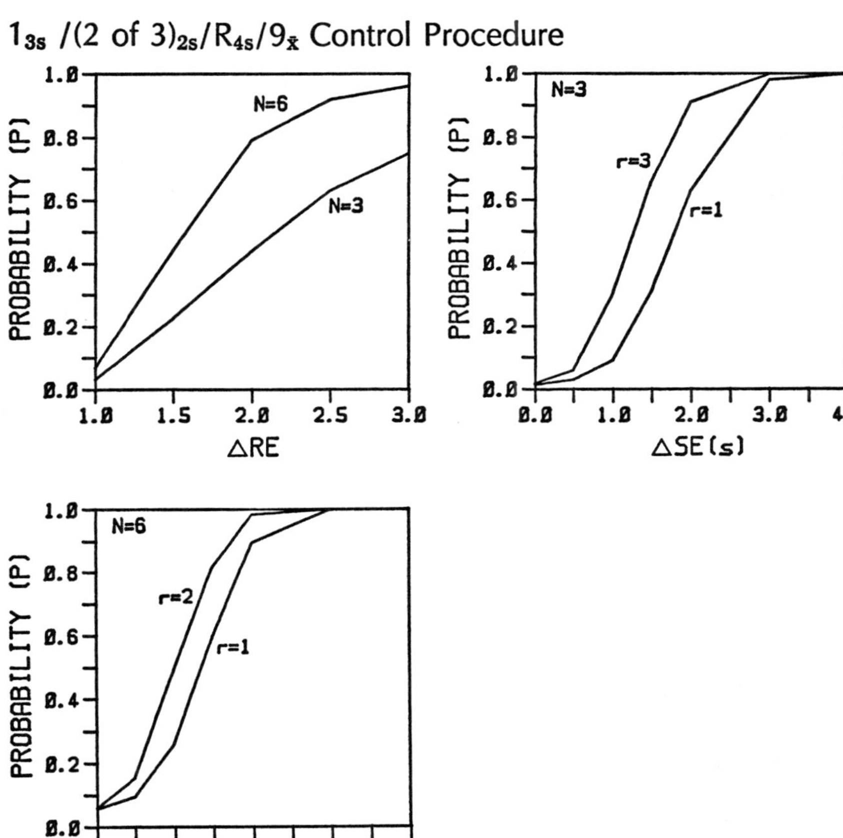

$1_{3s}/(2 \text{ of } 3)_{2s}/R_{4s}/12_{\bar{x}}$ Control Procedure

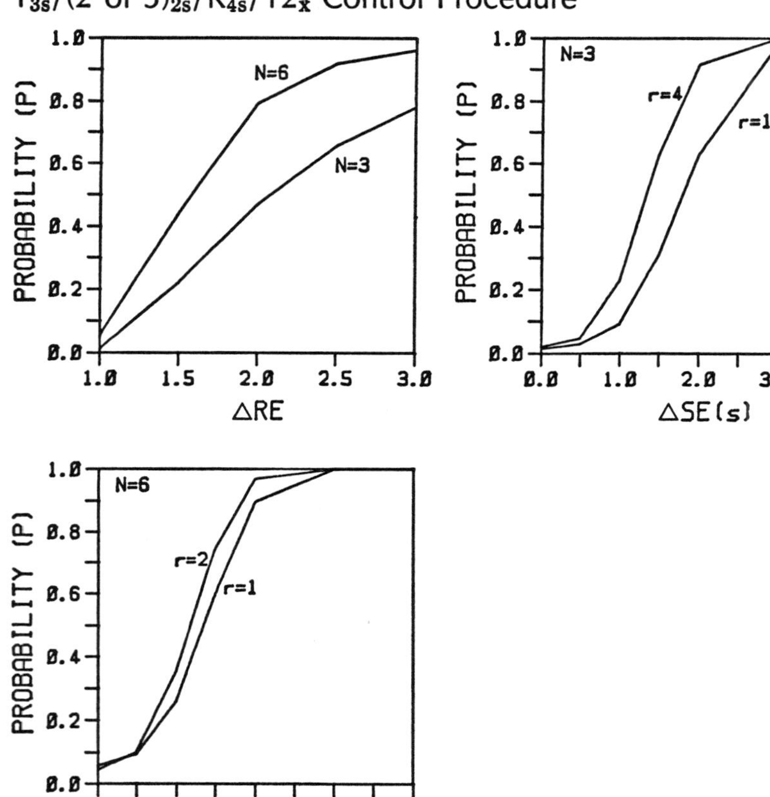

$1_{3s}/2_{2s}/R_{0.01}/4_{1s}/8_{\bar{x}}$ Control Procedure

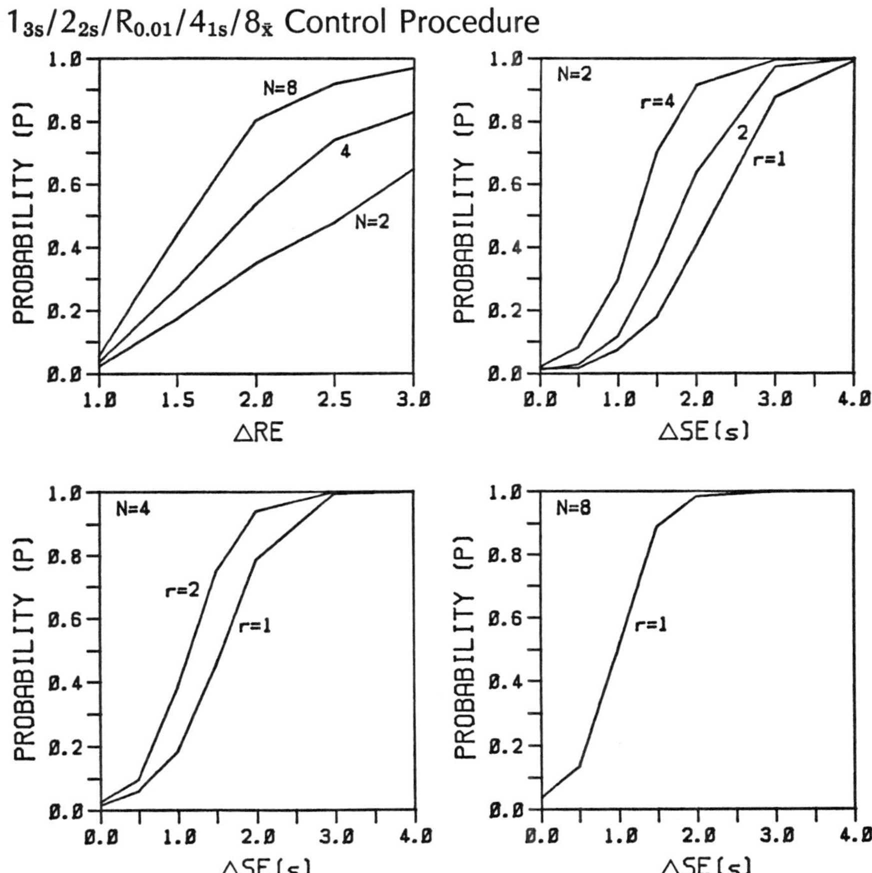

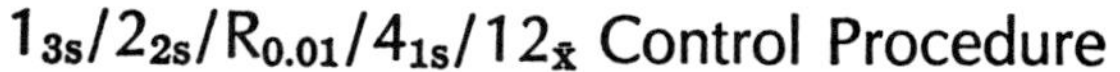

$1_{3s}/2_{2s}/R_{0.01}/4_{1s}/12_{\bar{x}}$ Control Procedure

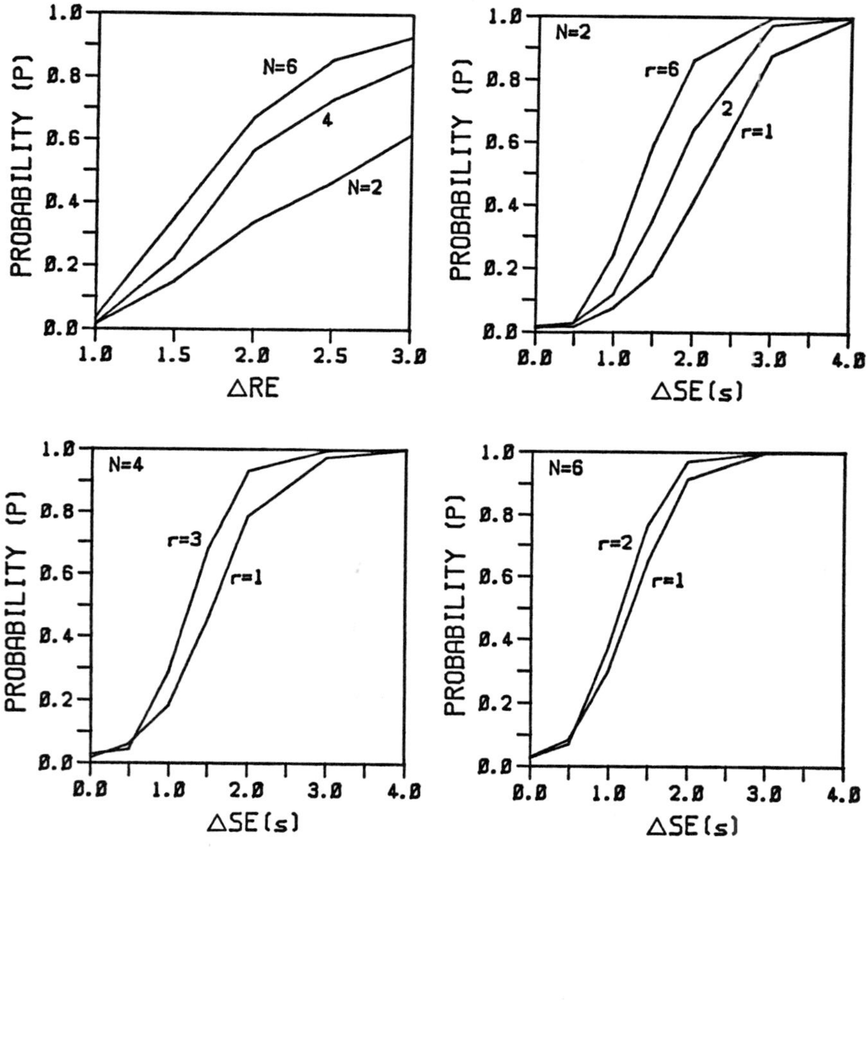

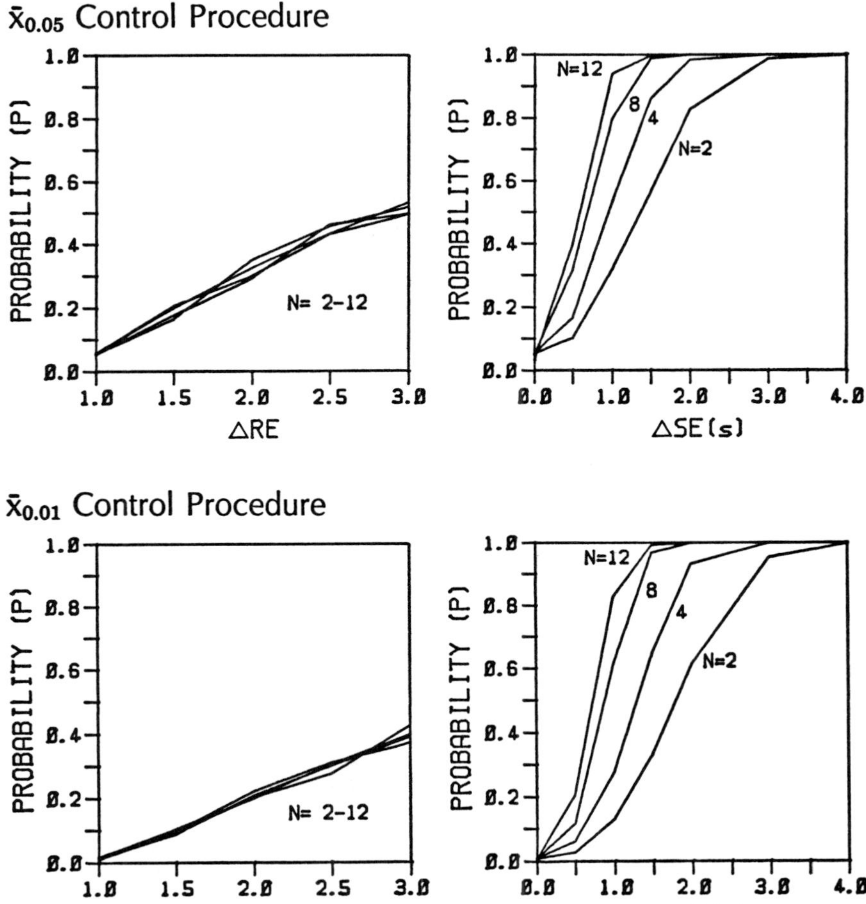
$\bar{x}_{0.05}$ Control Procedure
PROBABILITY (P)
1.0
0.8
0.6
0.4
0.2
0.0
N= 2-12
1.0 1.5 2.0 2.5 3.0
ΔRE
N=12
8
4
N=2
0.0 1.0 2.0 3.0 4.0
ΔSE(s)
$\bar{x}_{0.01}$ Control Procedure
PROBABILITY (P)
1.0
0.8
0.6
0.4
0.2
0.0
N= 2-12
1.0 1.5 2.0 2.5 3.0
ΔRE
N=12
8
4
N=2
0.0 1.0 2.0 3.0 4.0
ΔSE(s)

$R_{0.05}$ Control Procedure

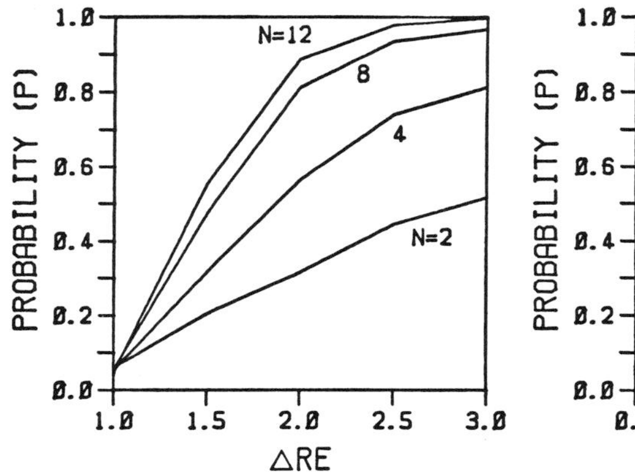

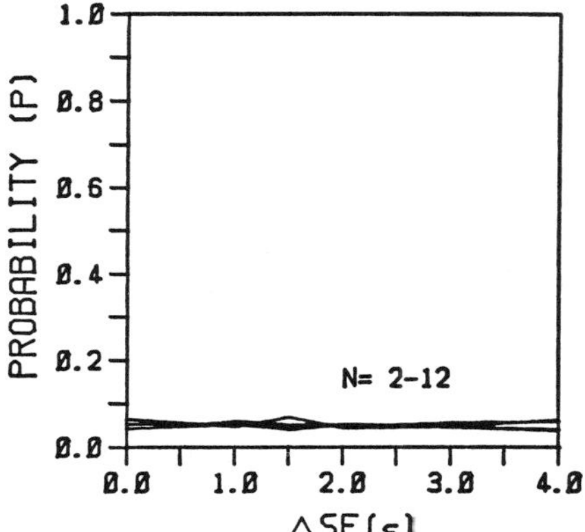

$R_{0.01}$ Control Procedure

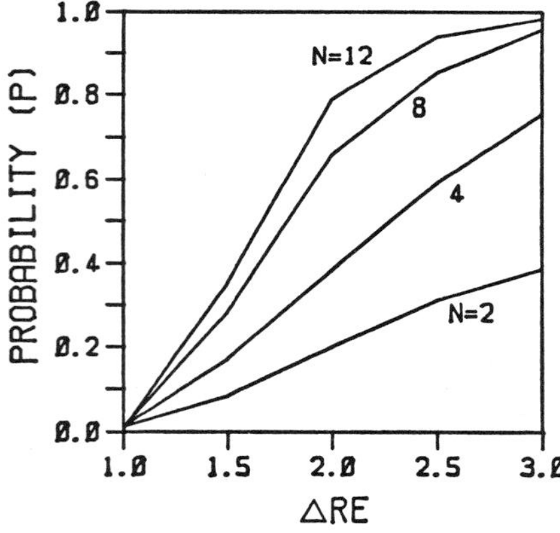

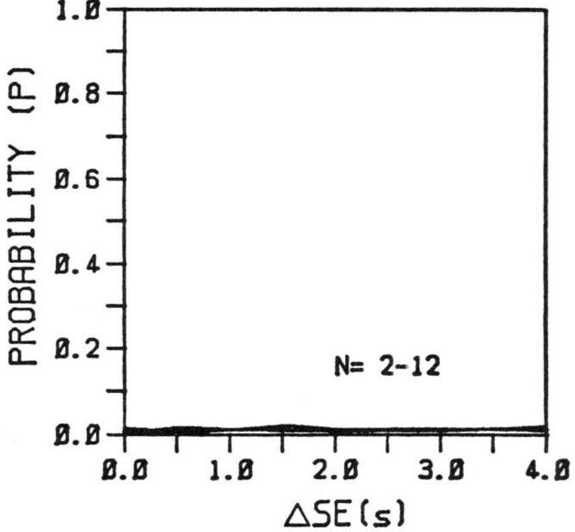

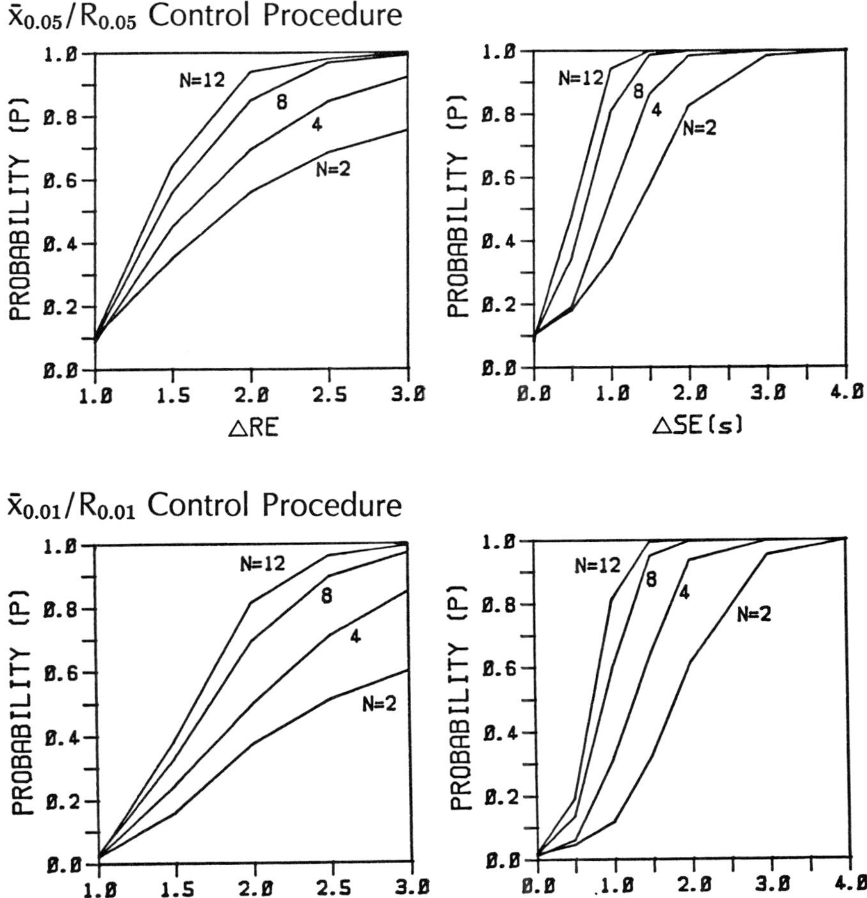
x̄0.05/R0.05 Control Procedure
PROBABILITY (P)
1.0
0.8
0.6
0.4
0.2
0.0
N=12
8
4
N=2
1.0 1.5 2.0 2.5 3.0
ΔRE
0.0 1.0 2.0 3.0 4.0
ΔSE(s)
x̄0.01/R0.01 Control Procedure
PROBABILITY (P)
N=12
8
4
N=2
ΔRE
ΔSE(s)

APPENDIX III

Spreadsheet Descriptions

Electronic spreadsheets, such as Lotus 1-2-3 (Lotus Development Corp., Cambridge, MA 02142), provide a convenient way for performing the average run length calculations described in Chapters 3 and 4 and for implementing the quality–productivity models described in Chapters 5 and 6. Descriptions of suitable spreadsheets are provided, using the convention that columns are identified by letters and rows are identified by numbers; e.g., C8 refers to the cell located in row 8 of column C.

For ARL calculations, it is convenient to have spreadsheets with 20, 40, and 100 rows. The example for 20 rows can be extended to provide those for 40 and 100 rows. For quality–productivity models, spreadsheets are described for batch and random access processes that are subject to intermittent and persistent errors.

Average Run Length (ARL) calculation (20 runs)

	-A-	-B-	-C-	-D-	-E-	-F-
1						
2						
3	RUN		PROPORTION	PROPORTION	CUMULATIVE	CALCULATED
4	NUMBER	Ped	OF ERRORS	OF ERRORS	PROPORTION	CONTRIBUTION
5	(or RUN	THIS	UNDETECTED	DETECTED	OF ERRORS	TO AVERAGE
6	LENGTH)	RUN	PRIOR TO RUN	THIS RUN	DETECTED	RUN LENGTH
7						
8	1		1	+B8*C8	+D8	+A8*D8
9	2		1-E8	+B9*C9	@SUM(D8..D9)	+A9*D9
10	3		1-E9	+B10*C10	@SUM(D8..D10)	+A10*D10
11	4		1-E10	+B11*C11	@SUM(D8..D11)	+A11*D11
12	5		1-E11	+B12*C12	@SUM(D8..D12)	+A12*D12
13	6		1-E12	+B13*C13	@SUM(D8..D13)	+A13*D13
14	7		1-E13	+B14*C14	@SUM(D8..D14)	+A14*D14
15	8		1-E14	+B15*C15	@SUM(D8..D15)	+A15*D15
16	9		1-E15	+B16*C16	@SUM(D8..D16)	+A16*D16
17	10		1-E16	+B17*C17	@SUM(D8..D17)	+A17*D17
18	11		1-E17	+B18*C18	@SUM(D8..D18)	+A18*D18
19	12		1-E18	+B19*C19	@SUM(D8..D19)	+A19*D19
20	13		1-E19	+B20*C20	@SUM(D8..D20)	+A20*D20
21	14		1-E20	+B21*C21	@SUM(D8..D21)	+A21*D21
22	15		1-E21	+B22*C22	@SUM(D8..D22)	+A22*D22
23	16		1-E22	+B23*C23	@SUM(D8..D23)	+A23*D23
24	17		1-E23	+B24*C24	@SUM(D8..D24)	+A24*D24
25	18		1-E24	+B25*C25	@SUM(D8..D25)	+A25*D25
26	19		1-E25	+B26*C26	@SUM(D8..D26)	+A26*D26
27	20		1-E26	+B27*C27	@SUM(D8..D27)	+A27*D27
28						
29				AVERAGE RUN LENGTH		@SUM(F8..F27)

Quality–productivity planning model for batch process with intermittent errors

MODEL:	BATCH PROCESS						
	INTERMITTENT ERRORS						
INPUT:	Instrument						
	Rules	1:2s					
	N	1.00					
	Ped	0.42			Rtr	1.00	
	Pfr	0.050			Rfr	1.00	
	C	1.00			Rfa	2.00	
	Sp	28.00			Rta	1.00	

OUTPUT:

Frequency (f)	0.00	0.01	0.02	0.05	0.10	0.20
Defect rate	0.00	0.01	0.01	0.03	0.06	0.12
CC-loss	0.07	0.07	0.07	0.07	0.07	0.07
TR-loss	0.00	0.00	0.01	0.02	0.04	0.08
FR-loss	0.05	0.05	0.05	0.04	0.04	0.04
FA-loss	0.00	0.01	0.02	0.05	0.11	0.22
TA-loss	0.00	0.01	0.01	0.02	0.05	0.08
Test yield	0.89	0.87	0.85	0.79	0.70	0.52

	-B-	-C-	-D-	-E-	-F-	-G-	-H-
1	BATCH PROCESS						
2	INTERMITTENT ERRORS						
3							
4	Instrument						
5	Rules	1:2s					
6	N	1					
7	Ped	0.42			Rtr	1	
8	Pfr	0.05			Rfr	1	
9	C	1			Rfa	2	
10	Sp	28			Rta	1	
11							
12							
13	Frequency (f)	0	0.01	0.02	0.05	0.1	0.2
14							
15	Defect rate	+C13*(1-C7)	+D13*(1-C7)	+E13*(1-C7)	+F13*(1-C7)	+G13*(1-C7)	+H13*(1-C7)
16	CC-loss	(C6+C9)/(C6+C9+C10)	(C6+C9)/(C6+C9+C10)	(C6+C9)/(C6+C9+C10)	(C6+C9)/(C6+C9+C10)	(C6+C9)/(C6+C9+C10)	(C6+C9)/(C6+C9+C10)
17	TR-loss	(C10/(C6+C9+C10))*G7*C13*C7	(C10/(C6+C9+C10))*G7*D13*C7	(C10/(C6+C9+C10))*G7*E13*C7	(C10/(C6+C9+C10))*G7*F13*C7	(C10/(C6+C9+C10))*G7*G13*C7	(C10/(C6+C9+C10))*G7*H13*C7
18	FR-loss	(C10/(C6+C9+C10))*G8*(1-C13)*C8	(C10/(C6+C9+C10))*G8*(1-D13)*C8	(C10/(C6+C9+C10))*G8*(1-E13)*C8	(C10/(C6+C9+C10))*G8*(1-F13)*C8	(C10/(C6+C9+C10))*G8*(1-G13)*C8	(C10/(C6+C9+C10))*G8*(1-H13)*C8
19	FA-loss	(C10/(C6+C9+C10))*G9*C13*(1-C7)	(C10/(C6+C9+C10))*G9*D13*(1-C7)	(C10/(C6+C9+C10))*G9*E13*(1-C7)	(C10/(C6+C9+C10))*G9*F13*(1-C7)	(C10/(C6+C9+C10))*G9*G13*(1-C7)	(C10/(C6+C9+C10))*G9*H13*(1-C7)
20	TA-loss	(C10/(C6+C9+C10))*G10*C13*(1-C7)*(1-C13)*(1-C8)	(C10/(C6+C9+C10))*G10*D13*(1-C7)*(1-D13)*(1-C8)	(C10/(C6+C9+C10))*G10*E13*(1-C7)*(1-E13)*(1-C8)	(C10/(C6+C9+C10))*G10*F13*(1-C7)*(1-F13)*(1-C8)	(C10/(C6+C9+C10))*G10*G13*(1-C7)*(1-G13)*(1-C8)	(C10/(C6+C9+C10))*G10*H13*(1-C7)*(1-H13)*(1-C8)
21	Test yield	1-@SUM(C16..C20)	1-@SUM(D16..D20)	1-@SUM(E16..E20)	1-@SUM(F16..F20)	1-@SUM(G16..G20)	1-@SUM(H16..H20)

Quality–productivity planning model for random access process with intermittent errors

```
MODEL:    RANDOM ACCESS
          INTERMITTENT ERRORS

INPUT:    Instrument
          Rules          1:2s
          N               1.00
          Ped             0.42            Rtr   1.00
          Pfr             0.050           Rfr   1.00
          C               1.00            Rfa   2.00
          Sp             28.00            Rta   1.00
```

OUTPUT:

Frequency (f)	0.00	0.01	0.02	0.05	0.10	0.20
Defect rate	0.00	0.01	0.01	0.03	0.06	0.12
CC-loss	0.07	0.07	0.07	0.07	0.07	0.07
TR-loss	0.00	0.00	0.00	0.00	0.00	0.00
FR-loss	0.00	0.00	0.00	0.00	0.00	0.00
FA-loss	0.00	0.01	0.02	0.05	0.11	0.22
TA-loss	0.00	0.01	0.01	0.02	0.05	0.08
Test yield	0.93	0.92	0.90	0.85	0.78	0.63

	-B-	-C-	-D-	-E-	-F-	-G-	-H-
1	RANDOM ACCESS						
2	INTERMITTENT ERRORS						
3							
4	Instrument						
5	Rules	1:2s					
6	N	1					
7	Ped	0.42			Rtr	1	
8	Pfr	0.05			Rfr	1	
9	C	1			Rfa	2	
10	Sp	28			Rta	1	
11							
12							
13	Frequency (f)	0	0.01	0.02	0.05	0.1	0.2
14							
15	Defect rate	+C13*(1-C7)	+D13*(1-C7)	+E13*(1-C7)	+F13*(1-C7)	+G13*(1-C7)	+H13*(1-C7)
16	CC-loss	(C6+C9)/(C6+C9+C10)	(C6+C9)/(C6+C9+C10)	(C6+C9)/(C6+C9+C10)	(C6+C9)/(C6+C9+C10)	(C6+C9)/(C6+C9+C10)	(C6+C9)/(C6+C9+C10)
17	TR-loss	(C6/(C6+C9+C10))*G7*C13*C7	(C6/(C6+C9+C10))*G7*D13*C7	(C6/(C6+C9+C10))*G7*E13*C7	(C6/(C6+C9+C10))*G7*F13*C7	(C6/(C6+C9+C10))*G7*G13*C7	(C6/(C6+C9+C10))*G7*H13*C7
18	FR-loss	(C6/(C6+C9+C10))*G8*(1-C13)*C8	(C6/(C6+C9+C10))*G8*(1-D13)*C8	(C6/(C6+C9+C10))*G8*(1-E13)*C8	(C6/(C6+C9+C10))*G8*(1-F13)*C8	(C6/(C6+C9+C10))*G8*(1-G13)*C8	(C6/(C6+C9+C10))*G8*(1-H13)*C8
19	FA-loss	(C10/(C6+C9+C10))*G9*C13*(1-C7)	(C10/(C6+C9+C10))*G9*D13*(1-C7)	(C10/(C6+C9+C10))*G9*E13*(1-C7)	(C10/(C6+C9+C10))*G9*F13*(1-C7)	(C10/(C6+C9+C10))*G9*G13*(1-C7)	(C10/(C6+C9+C10))*G9*H13*(1-C7)
20	TA-loss	(C10/(C6+C9+C10))*G10*C13*(1-C7)*(1-C13)*(1-C8)	(C10/(C6+C9+C10))*G10*D13*(1-C7)*(1-D13)*(1-C8)	(C10/(C6+C9+C10))*G10*E13*(1-C7)*(1-E13)*(1-C8)	(C10/(C6+C9+C10))*G10*F13*(1-C7)*(1-F13)*(1-C8)	(C10/(C6+C9+C10))*G10*G13*(1-C7)*(1-G13)*(1-C8)	(C10/(C6+C9+C10))*G10*H13*(1-C7)*(1-H13)*(1-C8)
21	Test yield	1-@SUM(C16..C20)	1-@SUM(D16..D20)	1-@SUM(E16..E20)	1-@SUM(F16..F20)	1-@SUM(G16..G20)	1-@SUM(H16..H20)

Quality–productivity planning model for batch process with persistent errors

```
MODEL:     BATCH PROCESS
           PERSISTENT ERRORS

INPUT:     Instrument
           Rules          1:2s
           N               1.00
           ARLr            2.38              Rtr   1.00
           ARLa           20.00              Rfr   1.00
           C               1.00              Rfa   2.00
           Sp             28.00              Rta   1.00

OUTPUT:
```

Frequency (f)	0.00	0.01	0.02	0.05	0.10	0.20
Defect rate	0.00	0.01	0.03	0.07	0.14	0.28
CC-loss	0.07	0.07	0.07	0.07	0.07	0.07
TR-loss	0.00	0.01	0.02	0.05	0.09	0.19
FR-loss	0.05	0.05	0.04	0.04	0.04	0.02
FA-loss	0.00	0.03	0.05	0.13	0.26	0.52
TA-loss	0.00	0.01	0.02	0.05	0.09	0.13
Test yield	0.89	0.84	0.80	0.66	0.45	0.08

	-B-	-C-	-D-	-E-	-F-	-G-	-H-
1	BATCH PROCESS						
2	PERSISTENT ERRORS						
3							
4	Instrument						
5	Rules	1:2s					
6	N	1					
7	ARLr	2.38			Rtr	1	
8	ARLa	20			Rfr	1	
9	C	1			Rfa	2	
10	Sp	28			Rta	1	
11							
12							
13	Frequency (f)	0	0.01	0.02	0.05	0.1	0.2
14							
15	Defect rate	+C13*(C7-1)	+D13*(C7-1)	+E13*(C7-1)	+F13*(C7-1)	+G13*(C7-1)	+H13*(C7-1)
16	CC-loss	(C6+C9)/(C6+C9+C10)	(C6+C9)/(C6+C9+C10)	(C6+C9)/(C6+C9+C10)	(C6+C9)/(C6+C9+C10)	(C6+C9)/(C6+C9+C10)	(C6+C9)/(C6+C9+C10)
17	TR-loss	(C10/(C6+C9+C10))*G7*C13	(C10/(C6+C9+C10))*G7*D13	(C10/(C6+C9+C10))*G7*E13	(C10/(C6+C9+C10))*G7*F13	(C10/(C6+C9+C10))*G7*G13	(C10/(C6+C9+C10))*G7*H13
18	FR-loss	(C10/(C6+C9+C10))*G8*(1-C7*C13)*(1/C8)	(C10/(C6+C9+C10))*G8*(1-C7*D13)*(1/C8)	(C10/(C6+C9+C10))*G8*(1-C7*E13)*(1/C8)	(C10/(C6+C9+C10))*G8*(1-C7*F13)*(1/C8)	(C10/(C6+C9+C10))*G8*(1-C7*G13)*(1/C8)	(C10/(C6+C9+C10))*G8*(1-C7*H13)*(1/C8)
19	FA-loss	(C10/(C6+C9+C10))*G9*C13*(C7-1)	(C10/(C6+C9+C10))*G9*D13*(C7-1)	(C10/(C6+C9+C10))*G9*E13*(C7-1)	(C10/(C6+C9+C10))*G9*F13*(C7-1)	(C10/(C6+C9+C10))*G9*G13*(C7-1)	(C10/(C6+C9+C10))*G9*H13*(C7-1)
20	TA-loss	(C10/(C6+C9+C10))*G10*C13*(C7-1)*(1-C7*C13)*(1-(1/C8))	(C10/(C6+C9+C10))*G10*D13*(C7-1)*(1-C7*D13)*(1-(1/C8))	(C10/(C6+C9+C10))*G10*E13*(C7-1)*(1-C7*E13)*(1-(1/C8))	(C10/(C6+C9+C10))*G10*F13*(C7-1)*(1-C7*F13)*(1-(1/C8))	(C10/(C6+C9+C10))*G10*G13*(C7-1)*(1-C7*G13)*(1-(1/C8))	(C10/(C6+C9+C10))*G10*H13*(C7-1)*(1-C7*H13)*(1-(1/C8))
21	Test yield	1-@SUM(C16..C20)	1-@SUM(D16..D20)	1-@SUM(E16..E20)	1-@SUM(F16..F20)	1-@SUM(G16..G20)	1-@SUM(H16..H20)

Quality–productivity planning model for random access process with persistent errors

MODEL: RANDOM ACCESS
PERSISTENT ERRORS

INPUT: Instrument

Rules	1:2s		
N	1.00		
ARLr	2.38	Rtr	1.00
ARLa	20.00	Rfr	1.00
C	1.00	Rfa	2.00
Sp	28.00	Rta	1.00

OUTPUT:

Frequency (f)	0.00	0.01	0.02	0.05	0.10	0.20
Defect rate	0.00	0.01	0.03	0.07	0.14	0.28
CC-loss	0.07	0.07	0.07	0.07	0.07	0.07
TR-loss	0.00	0.00	0.00	0.00	0.00	0.01
FR-loss	0.00	0.00	0.00	0.00	0.00	0.00
FA-loss	0.00	0.03	0.05	0.13	0.26	0.52
TA-loss	0.00	0.01	0.02	0.05	0.09	0.13
Test yield	0.93	0.89	0.86	0.75	0.58	0.28

	-B-	-C-	-D-	-E-	-F-	-G-	-H-
1	RANDOM ACCESS						
2	PERSISTENT ERRORS						
3							
4	Instrument						
5	Rules	1:2s					
6	N	1					
7	ARLr	2.38			Rtr	1	
8	ARLa	20			Rfr	1	
9	C	1			Rfa	2	
10	Sp	28			Rta	1	
11							
12							
13	Frequency (f)	0	0.01	0.02	0.05	0.1	0.2
14							
15	Defect rate	+C13*(C7-1)	+D13*(C7-1)	+E13*(C7-1)	+F13*(C7-1)	+G13*(C7-1)	+H13*(C7-1)
16	CC-loss	(C6+C9)/(C6+C9+C 10)	(C6+C9)/(C6+C9+C 10)	(C6+C9)/(C6+C9+C 10)	(C6+C9)/(C6+C9+C 10)	(C6+C9)/(C6+C9+C 10)	(C6+C9)/(C6+C9+C 10)
17	TR-loss	(C6/(C6+C9+C10)) *G7*C13	(C6/(C6+C9+C10)) *G7*D13	(C6/(C6+C9+C10)) *G7*E13	(C6/(C6+C9+C10)) *G7*F13	(C6/(C6+C9+C10)) *G7*G13	(C6/(C6+C9+C10)) *G7*H13
18	FR-loss	(C6/(C6+C9+C10)) *G8*(1-C7*C13)*(1/C8)	(C6/(C6+C9+C10)) *G8*(1-C7*D13)*(1/C8)	(C6/(C6+C9+C10)) *G8*(1-C7*E13)*(1/C8)	(C6/(C6+C9+C10)) *G8*(1-C7*F13)*(1/C8)	(C6/(C6+C9+C10)) *G8*(1-C7*G13)*(1/C8)	(C6/(C6+C9+C10)) *G8*(1-C7*H13)*(1/C8)
19	FA-loss	(C10/(C6+C9+C10))*G9*C13*(C7-1)	(C10/(C6+C9+C10))*G9*D13*(C7-1)	(C10/(C6+C9+C10))*G9*E13*(C7-1)	(C10/(C6+C9+C10))*G9*F13*(C7-1)	(C10/(C6+C9+C10))*G9*G13*(C7-1)	(C10/(C6+C9+C10))*G9*H13*(C7-1)
20	TA-loss	(C10/(C6+C9+C10))*G10*C13*(C7-1) *(1-C7*C13)*(1-(1/C8))	(C10/(C6+C9+C10))*G10*D13*(C7-1) *(1-C7*D13)*(1-(1/C8))	(C10/(C6+C9+C10))*G10*E13*(C7-1) *(1-C7*E13)*(1-(1/C8))	(C10/(C6+C9+C10))*G10*F13*(C7-1) *(1-C7*F13)*(1-(1/C8))	(C10/(C6+C9+C10))*G10*G13*(C7-1) *(1-C7*G13)*(1-(1/C8))	(C10/(C6+C9+C10))*G10*H13*(C7-1) *(1-C7*H13)*(1-(1/C8))
21	Test yield	1-@SUM(C16..C20)	1-@SUM(D16..D20)	1-@SUM(E16..E20)	1-@SUM(F16..F20)	1-@SUM(G16..G20)	1-@SUM(H16..H20)

INDEX